Understanding MRI

Understanding MRI

Jeffrey H. Newhouse, M.D.
Professor of Radiology, College of Physicians and Surgeons
of Columbia University; Director of Abdominal Radiology
and Body Imaging, Columbia-Presbyterian Medical Center,
New York, New York

Jonathan I. Wiener, M.D.
Assistant Clinical Professor of Radiology, University of
Miami School of Medicine; Director of MRI, Boca Raton
Community Hospital, Boca Raton, Florida

Little, Brown and Company
Boston/Toronto/London

To our parents

Contents

Preface

This short book is an attempt to explain some of the physical processes that underlie nuclear magnetic resonance (NMR) imaging, a technology now more often referred to as magnetic resonance imaging, or MRI. Both of us are radiologists, and neither has had advanced training in physics or mathematics. We have had an experience that many radiologists and other practitioners in the field of imaging may have shared, which is that explanations of the physical principles of MRI are either too short to satisfy our curiosity, too burdened with mathematics for us to unravel, or couched in terms familiar only to physicists. We have, therefore, tried to write a book that we wish we had had when we started learning about MRI.

We have assumed that the reader has no more knowledge of physics than might reasonably be remembered by a radiologist who trained in the pre-MRI era and who may have forgotten a great deal of the physics he or she did know. We also have assumed that the reader may no longer be facile with mathematics, and have therefore tried to keep formulas to a minimum. And because the reader may not be familiar with much of the terminology of physics, we have attempted either to avoid or to explain it. Finally, we have assumed that the reader wishes to acquaint himself or herself with a particular scope of MRI knowledge.

Specifically, we present some of the most basic underlying phenomena upon which MRI depends and explain those phenomena that are pertinent to the operation of an MRI device. The readers of this book will be able to understand what an MR image represents, will be able to understand the major parameters that need to be adjusted when operating an MRI machine, and will be sufficiently familiar with the operation of the machine and its underlying physical principles to think about variations in imaging technique and machine operation for themselves.

In the description of the physical phenomena, we could have chosen to describe a classic mechanical model or a quantum mechanical one. Although, beyond a certain level of sophistication, the quantum model may more accurately describe certain phenomena, the classic model works equally well for the concepts presented in this book, and since we think that this model might be easier for most of our readers to comprehend, we have chosen to use it.

J.H.N.
J.I.W.

Acknowledgments

We are extremely grateful for the efforts of those whose help made this volume possible. The manuscript was reviewed and much improved by Edward Nickoloff. Madeline Cannella and Anna Calderin remained patient and good-humored while typing the countless drafts. Brian Sota drew and patiently revised all of the diagrams. Jane Licht made the many steps of publication both efficient and pleasurable. We deeply appreciate their contributions.

Understanding MRI

Introduction

Even before we begin to consider the most basic elements of NMR scanning, it might be useful to have an overview of the primary things an NMR imaging device does.

Figure I-1 is an extremely simple representation of what goes on. In brief, the body part to be examined is placed in a strong magnetic field, and is also subjected to short pulses of radio frequency energy that come from a nearby antenna. These two effects cause the body tissue to give off radio frequency signal of its own. The signal is picked up by an antenna and fed into a computer, which can generate an image from the information contained in this signal.

We do not intend to describe all of the steps in this process in equal detail. What we will do is present the very basics of the phenomena that occur to and within body tissues, how they are recorded, how they are turned into an image, and how they can be controlled and understood by the MRI operator.

Since we have assumed that the reader has relatively little background in physics or MR, we will begin the discussion with certain concepts whose application to imaging may not be immediately apparent, but which are necessary to comprehend in order to make sense of the discussion that follows. The first of these concepts is that of the vector.

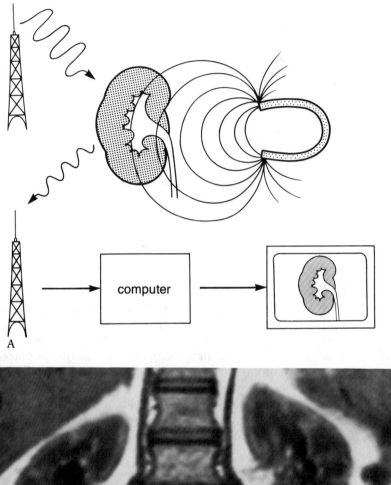

B

FIGURE I-1.

A. The MRI process, extremely oversimplified. The structure to be imaged (shown here as a kidney) rests in a magnetic field. It receives radio frequency signal from an antenna, and subsequently emits radio frequency signal of a lower magnitude. This emitted signal interacts with another antenna (frequently the same antenna is used for both), undergoes extensive computer-controlled transformations, and is ultimately used to form an image. B. MRI of kidneys.

CHAPTER *1*

Vectors

A *vector* is a mathematic tool that scientists use to represent certain physical phenomena. Vectors are frequently used in the description of nuclear magnetic resonance (NMR), so it is necessary to become familiar with them.

A vector represents a quantity with both magnitude and direction. For example, a physical force may be represented by a vector. Such a force is represented by the drawing in Fig. 1-1. The force is represented by the arrow; it is pushing on the object represented by the cube. The usual convention is to draw a vector as an arrow, as we have done in this

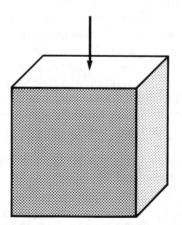

FIGURE 1-1.
A simple vector. A force pushing downward on the solid cube can be represented by an arrow, whose length indicates the magnitude of the force and whose direction indicates the force's direction.

3

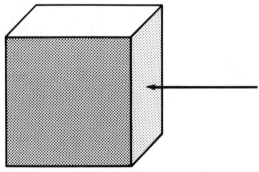

FIGURE 1-2.
Another vector. A force, twice as large as the one seen in Fig. 1-1, is represented by an arrow twice as long. The direction of the force is to the left.

case. The arrow, of course, indicates a direction; it is also
important to note that the *quantity* of the force is directly
proportional to the length of the arrow. The vector in Fig. 1-
2 depicts another force; it is pushing twice as hard on the
object, and is pushing in another direction.

Vectors are not only used to describe physical forces. They
may, for example, describe magnetic fields, and it is in this
context that we will ultimately be using them. For the moment, however, the important ideas to retain are that a vector is conventionally drawn as an arrow, the quantity of the
phenomenon that it depicts is represented by the length of
the arrow, and the direction of the phenomenon is represented by the direction of the arrow.

To describe vectors that can point in any direction in
space, we need a three-dimensional coordinate system. One
that we might use is depicted in Fig. 1-3; this one is, for
all practical purposes, identical to the one scientists use to
describe NMR phenomena. In this system, the Z direction is
the vertical axis within the plane of the page, the X direction
is the horizontal axis within the plane of the page, and the
Y axis is the axis perpendicular to the plane of the page. The
plane in which the X and Y axes exist—that is, the plane
perpendicular to the Z axis—is known as the XY plane, or
the transverse plane.

A vector's magnitude and direction can be represented in
this system, as shown in Fig. 1-4. In it, vector A is seen
pointing in the positive direction along the Z axis. The vector has a magnitude, which, as we have pointed out earlier,
is directly proportional to the length of the arrow. Another

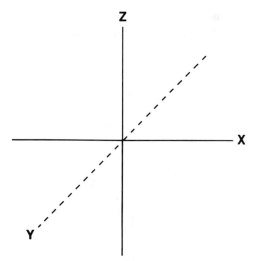

FIGURE 1-3.
Three-dimensional coordinate system. These axes are a commonly used background against which to describe magnetic fields. The Z axis, by convention, represents the direction of the main magnetic field in which an NMR experiment is done. The X and Y axes are within a plane (the "transverse" plane) that is perpendicular to the Z axis.

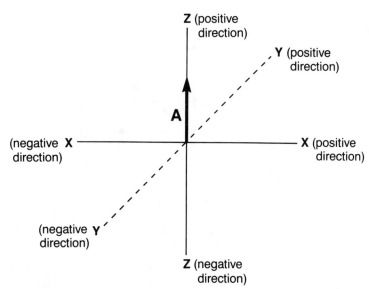

FIGURE 1-4.
A vector, labeled A, in the three-dimensional coordinate system. The vector points in the positive Z direction and its magnitude is represented by the length of the arrow.

vector, vector B, in Fig. 1-5, is in the Z axis, but is in the negative Z direction, and has an absolute magnitude proportional to its length.

In Fig. 1-6, vector M is drawn. It does not lie directly along

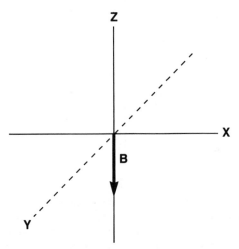

FIGURE 1-5.
Another vector, labeled B. This, too, is in the Z axis but points in the negative direction.

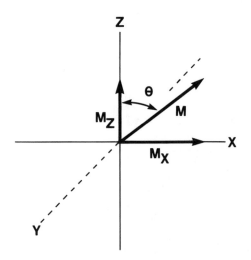

FIGURE 1-6.
A vector labeled M. This vector lies in the plane that contains the X and Z axes; its direction is different from the Z axis by the angle θ. The vector can be resolved into components M_z and M_x, which are in the Z and X directions, respectively. If M_z and M_x represented independent entities, their sum would be identical to, and indistinguishable from, vector M. Alternatively, an entity described by the vector M could equally well be described by the simultaneous vectors M_z and M_x.

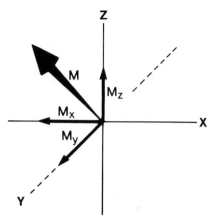

FIGURE 1-7.
Another vector, labeled M. This one has components in the Z, X, and Y axes. As in the previous example, if the components of the X, Y, and Z vectors (M_x, M_y, and M_z, respectively) were added together, they would reconstitute the original vector.

any axis, but our principal rules still hold: Its direction is depicted by the direction of the arrow and its magnitude (M) by the length of the arrow. The vector makes an angle θ with the X axis.

Vector M may be divided into certain components. It can be said to have a magnitude in the X direction (seen in Fig. 1-6 as M_x) and a magnitude in the Z direction (seen in Fig. 1-6 as M_z). It has no magnitude in the Y direction. This division of the vector into components is important. In our system, the two components—that is, the vector along the X axis and the vector along the Z axis—would, if added together, produce the original vector. For our purposes, the components and the original vector can be thought of as the same; that is, the phenomenon depicted by the original vector can also be thought of as the two components acting together. Conversely, two original vectors that were exactly like the two components may also be thought of as a single vector identical to our original one.

Let us examine one more situation. In Fig. 1-7, vector M has magnitude in all three axes. As with the previous example, the original vector M can be quite accurately thought of as being the same as the combination of the component vectors; that is, M_x, M_y, and M_z, when added together, are the same as vector M.

Throughout this book vectors are used frequently to describe magnetic fields, each of which has a specific magnitude (no half puns intended; the magnitude of a magnetic field is the strength of that field) and a direction.

CHAPTER 2

Magnets and Magnetic Fields

Magnets produce magnetic fields; magnetic fields, in turn, can be produced by either permanent magnets or electric currents flowing in conductors, or both. Figure 2-1 shows a simple permanent magnet with a north and south pole; the magnetic field it produces is indicated by the curved lines.

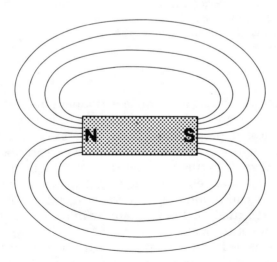

FIGURE 2-1.
Simple bar magnet. The magnetic field produced by this magnet is depicted by the curved lines. At any point in space, the strength of the field is proportional to the closeness of the lines, and the direction of the field is indicated by the direction of the lines.

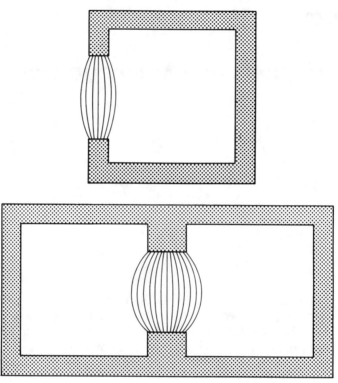

FIGURE 2-2.
Other configurations of permanent magnets. Again, the strength of the magnetic field at any point is indicated by the closeness of the lines, and the direction of the field by the direction of the lines.

Figure 2-2 reveals two simple permanent magnets; as in Fig. 2-1, the magnetic field is represented by multiple lines whose closeness is proportional to the strength of the field at any point. Figure 2-3 shows a straight wire carrying a current; the current in this wire generates a magnetic field whose lines of flux are circular. Figure 2-4 demonstrates a solenoidal wire coil conducting a current; again, the magnetic field is represented in this diagram by lines within and outside the core of the coil.

It is not within the scope of this text to describe the details of the various kinds of magnets. Figure 2-2 is similar to forms of permanent magnets currently in use; certainly, other configurations of permanent magnets have been used to produce images. Figure 2-4 represents a common configuration of an electromagnet, that is, a magnet in which the magnetic field is produced by flowing current rather than by

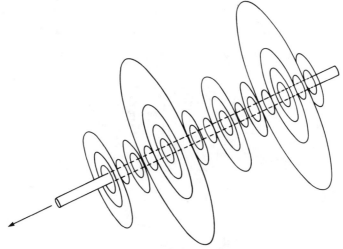

FIGURE 2-3.
A straight wire conducting a current whose direction is indicated by the arrow. The circles in the space around the wire represent the magnet field's lines of flux that the flowing current causes.

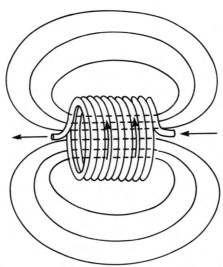

FIGURE 2-4.
Air-cored solenoidal electromagnet. The direction of the current flowing along the coiled wire is shown by the arrows, and the resultant magnetic field is demonstrated by the curved lines. Note that within the coil of the magnet, the lines are roughly parallel and equidistant. Such a magnet can be designed so that the magnetic field within its bore is relatively homogeneous.

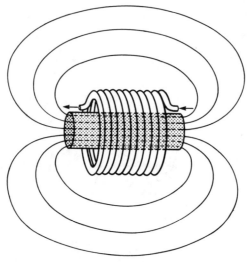

FIGURE 2-5.
Iron-cored solenoidal electromagnet. If an iron bar, rather than air, occupies the central bore of the magnet, and the configuration of the coil and of the current through it is the same as in an air-cored magnet, the field within the iron bar will be stronger than the field within the bore of an air-cored magnet.

a permanent magnet. Electromagnets may have air in the core, as in this case, or iron in the core, as in Fig. 2-5. The coils of wire used to make an electromagnet either may be approximately at room temperature, in which case the electromagnet is termed a *resistive magnet*, or the magnet may be supercooled; that is, one which is cooled by some means to a sufficiently low temperature that current flows in the wire without encountering any resistance.

A wire that can conduct electricity without significant resistance is known as a *superconductor*; most magnets currently used for clinical imaging today are superconducting. The standard method for cooling the wire windings is to enclose the entire magnet in a jacket of liquid helium, which in turn is enclosed in a jacket of liquid nitrogen; the temperature of the magnet is brought quite close to absolute zero (0 degrees Kelvin), which is necessary for superconductivity to appear.

Current research has produced substances that display superconductivity at ever higher temperatures and these substances may eventually be used to create superconducting imaging magnets. Resistive magnets have been used for clinical imaging as well. They are cheaper to construct than superconducting magnets are, but the magnetic fields of resistive magnets are relatively low, they require large amounts of current, and they generate a considerable amount of heat. Most magnetic resonance imaging (MRI) devices presently being built do not use resistive magnets.

A few MRI devices are constructed using permanent magnets; these have the advantage of having low operating costs, but are restricted to moderately low fields and are very heavy.

We now need to discuss some of the features of the magnetic field generated by the magnet. First of all, one should note by looking at Figs. 1-3, 2-2, and 2-5 that if an iron-core magnet is used (either permanent or electromagnetic), the magnetic lines of flux run from the north pole to the south pole. In an air-cored electromagnet, such as that in Fig. 2-4, there is no north or south pole per se; rather, the magnetic lines of flux run in continuous loops through the core of the magnet and around the outside of the magnet. The magnetic field outside the imaging core of the magnet is known as the "fringe field." It is this magnetic field that produces potential danger for personnel who must work near the magnet, since the field may affect cardiac pacemakers, accelerate iron objects within it, and so forth. It is in order to contain this field that magnetic shielding devices are used.

Let us assume a convention in which the magnetic lines of force denote the field. First of all, the strength of the field deserves some attention. The field is stronger in areas in which the magnetic field lines are drawn closer together (see Figs. 2-1 through 2-5). The units of strength of the field are the *gauss* or *Tesla*; 10,000 gauss are equal to 1 Tesla. To provide a standard of comparison, the earth's magnetic field, at least in the midlatitudes, is approximately 0.6 gauss. The magnetic field near a small permanent magnet of the type usually used to attach children's drawings to refrigerator doors may be several hundred gauss; the strongest of toy magnets may generate fields as high as a Tesla or so, at least in small regions near the poles of the magnet.

For imaging, the magnetic field must be as homogeneous as possible; that is, within the volume occupied by the imaged patient, the field must be as close as possible to a constant strength when measured at various places within the volume. The lines in Fig. 2-6 describe a magnetic field; these

FIGURE 2-6.
Lines of flux denoting a homogeneous magnetic field. The strength of the field is the same from place to place within it.

lines might, for example, represent the magnetic field seen within the core of the magnet depicted in Fig. 2-4. Notice that the lines are straight and parallel. Since the magnetic field strength is proportional to the closeness of the lines, in this case, the magnetic field is exactly the same strength wherever it is measured. But this is an ideal situation; no one has ever been able to build a magnet that produces a field of absolute homogeneity. Instead, the field really looks more like that depicted in Fig. 2-7. Here, notice that in some places the magnetic lines of flux are closer together than they are in others; in regions where the lines are close together, the field is stronger than it is elsewhere. There are a number of reasons why these inhomogeneities should be reduced as much as possible for MRI; we mention some of these later. For the moment, it should be noted that the field inhomogeneities are less than 10 parts per million in the imaging volume of a high-quality magnet; the volume in which these limitations are specified is usually a 35- to 40-

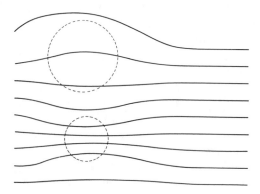

FIGURE 2-7.
Lines of flux of an inhomogeneous magnetic field. Where the lines are close together (as in the area within the lower dotted circle), the field is relatively strong; where they are far apart (upper dotted circle), the field is relatively weak.

cm sphere, which is the space occupied by the structures being imaged.

All real magnets, no matter how carefully they are designed and constructed, produce fields with some degree of inhomogeneity. The inhomogeneity can be diminished (but not eliminated) by a process called *shimming.* Shimming can be accomplished by placing within the magnet small pieces of iron or other ferromagnetic material that can locally alter the direction of the magnetic lines of flux slightly. If the shims are placed correctly, their effects can be used to diminish the inhomogeneity of the field. This is called *passive shimming.* Alternatively, the magnetic field may be altered slightly by placing wire coils within it and passing current through them; careful manipulation of the shape, position, and current of these coils may also diminish local inhomogeneity. This is called *active shimming.*

Figures 2-6 and 2-7 reveal ideal (without inhomogeneities) and real magnetic fields. They are without gradients; that is, if one travels over a considerable distance within the field, one does not encounter a large and consistent change in overall magnetic field strength (especially if one ignores the minor local variations depicted in Fig. 2-7). Figure 2-8, on

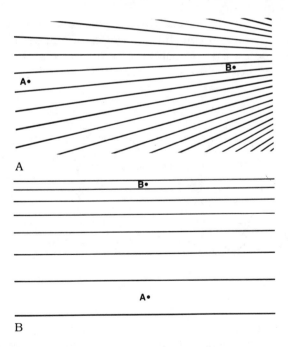

FIGURE 2-8.
Magnetic fields with gradients. A. The magnetic field gets stronger as one travels from left to right; the field is stronger at point B than at point A. B. The gradient is from the bottom to the top; again, the field is stronger at point B than at point A.

the other hand, reveals magnetic fields that do display field strength gradients; as one goes from point A to point B, one encounters an increase in overall field strength. A *magnetic gradient*, then, is a condition in which the strength varies from place to place within the field. Within the region of the magnet used for imaging, magnetic field gradients are usually made to be *linear*; that is, there is a linear and constant relationship between the distance in a particular direction and the change of magnetic field associated with that distance.

Magnetic field strength gradients—referred to, for short, as magnetic gradients or merely as gradients—are frequently used in MRI. Typically, a magnet produces a field without a gradient, and then wire coils are placed within the magnet's bore. When current is allowed to flow through these coils, they act as magnets within magnets, and shape the overall magnetic field to have a particular gradient. Figure 2-9 depicts such a situation: The main magnet has created a field and current is passing through the coil; a field with a gradient has been produced. The shape and orientation of the gradient coils are quite variable, so the direction and strength of the magnetic field gradient within the magnet are quite variable as well.

We have introduced the concept of vectors, and described briefly some of the characteristics of magnetic fields, and at this point wish to combine some aspects of the two. Since a magnetic field has a magnitude and a direction, it can be

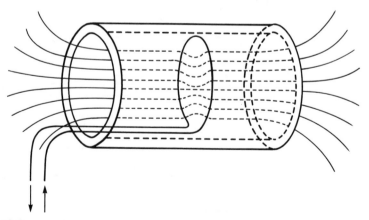

FIGURE 2-9.
Air-cored solenoidal magnet. The hollow cylinder contains the windings of a solenoidal electromagnet. A single loop of wire in the core of the magnet has a current flowing within it, as indicated by the arrows, and causes local gradients in the magnetic field.

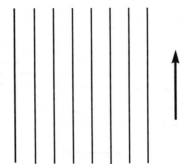

FIGURE 2-10.
A vector representing a magnetic field. The lines of flux of the field are parallel to the vector, and the strength of the field is proportional to the vector's length.

represented as a vector. The magnetic field represented in Fig. 2-6 could also be represented by the vector in Fig. 2-10; as with other vectors, the length of the arrow is proportional to the strength of the magnetic field and its direction is parallel to the magnetic flux lines. Figure 2-11 demonstrates another configuration of a magnetic field and its vector.

Now remember that a vector can describe *any* phenomenon that has a magnitude and a direction; therefore, a magnetic field *gradient* can also be described as a vector. Figure 2-12 depicts magnetic fields that have gradients; the gradients are indicated by arrows. By convention, the direction of the arrow is the direction of increasing magnetic field; the length of the arrow describes the magnitude of the gradient.

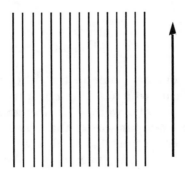

FIGURE 2-11.
The parallel lines again denoting the lines of flux of the field and the adjacent arrow; the vector describing the field. Note that the strength of the field, and hence the length of the vector, is greater here than in Fig. 2-10.

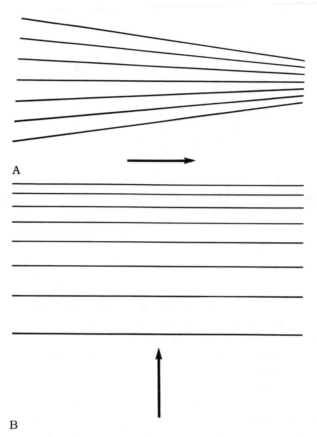

A

B

FIGURE 2-12.
Vectors representing the magnetic field gradients (*not* the fields themselves; these are represented by the other lines). A. The gradient is oriented from left to right and has a magnitude proportional to the length of the arrow. B. The gradient goes from the bottom to the top of the image and, again, is represented by the direction and length of the vector arrow.

The units for the magnitude of a vector describing a magnetic field gradient would be milliTesla (or gauss) per centimeter.

We now consider some of the other characteristics of a magnetic field, which are important to consider for the safety of those who work within or near such fields. It is certainly common knowledge that a magnetic field may exert a force on certain metal (specifically ferromagnetic) objects or materials, and that magnets small enough to be placed entirely within other magnetic fields may be subjected to particularly strong forces. These phenomena are not particularly important for NMR imaging, but do come into play when matters of safety around large magnets are concerned.

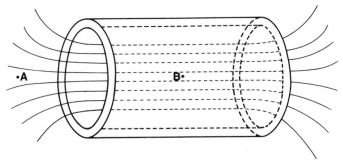

FIGURE 2-13.
At point A, the field is weaker than at point B, but there is a gradient (at point A) which could be denoted as an arrow pointing from left to right, whereas at point B there is no gradient. A ferromagnetic object at point A will experience a linear force, but no such force would be experienced by an object at point B. The force at point A would be proportional to the strength of the gradient as well as the strength of the field. A ferromagnetic object that could be induced to have a north pole and south pole would experience a *torque* at *both* point A and point B. The torque would tend to rotate the object so that its long axis is parallel to the field in either site, and the strength of the torque would be proportional to the strength of the field, *not* to the strength of the gradient, at either point.

First of all, it should be noted that a linear force may or may not be exerted by a magnetic field on a ferromagnetic object. In general, a ferromagnetic object will experience such a force if it exists within a magnetic field that has a gradient; if it does, it will be pulled in a direction toward the stronger field. If the field has no gradient, a ferromagnetic object will not experience any linear force. Figure 2-13, which is like Fig. 2-9, represents the magnetic field produced by a large solenoidal coil of the type commonly used in MRI devices. A ferromagnetic object placed at point A will be pulled toward the center of the magnet's bore, that is, up the magnetic field gradient. But an object within the bore, where there is no gradient, will not experience any force.

Another effect that magnetic fields have on ferromagnetic objects is to subject them to a *torque*, that is, a rotational force. In general, a ferromagnetic object that has one axis longer than the other (for example, a bar of steel) will experience a torque such that its long axis will be forced toward alignment with the magnetic flux lines. This torque is proportional to the strength of the field rather than to the strength of gradient. Therefore, in Fig. 2-13 the torque would be greatest where the linear force is least, that is, in the center of the magnet's bore at point B.

CHAPTER 3

Electromagnetic Induction and Electromagnetic Waves

ELECTROMAGNETIC INDUCTION

We mentioned earlier that a current flowing through a wire can produce a magnetic field. Now we present the converse notion. Under certain circumstances, a magnetic field can be used to induce a voltage, and hence produce current. For this to happen, the lines of flux of the magnetic field must move across the axis of the wire in which the current is to be induced. This can be done by either moving a wire through a magnetic field (Fig. 3-1) or moving the lines of flux of the magnetic field across the wire. This latter may be accom-

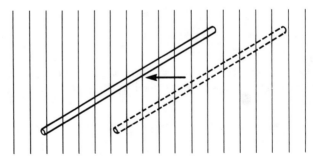

FIGURE 3-1.
A piece of wire moving sideways through a magnetic field. If the direction of motion is such that the wire moves across lines of flux, a voltage will be induced in the wire.

plished in several ways; one might do an experiment in
which a wire was held stationary and a magnet was moved
in the proximity of the wire (Fig. 3-2) or one might construct
an electromagnet with an adjacent wire such as that seen in
Fig. 3-3. If the strength of the field generated by the electromagnet were changed (by increasing or decreasing the current in its coils), the flux lines of the magnet's magnetic field
would change in position. As the flux lines cross the adjacent
wire, they would induce a current in it. This last phenomenon—that is, the induction of a voltage and hence a current
in a wire by alterations in the strenth of a magnetic field
near the wire—is central to the operation of an NMR imaging device.

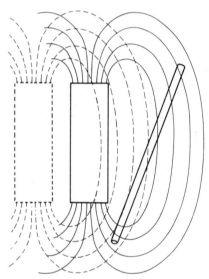

FIGURE 3-2.
The wire is stationary but the lines of flux of the magnetic field move as the
magnet moves. A voltage will be induced in the wire.

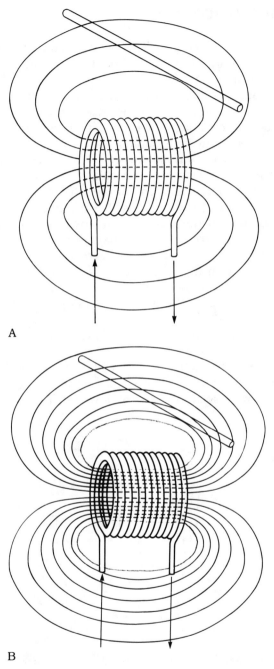

A

B

FIGURE 3-3.
A wire in the field of a solenoidal magnet. A. The current in the coil is weaker
than in B. B. As the current increases, the magnetic lines of flux move closer
together and closer to the magnet. As they move through the wire, they will
cause a voltage to be induced in the wire.

ELECTROMAGNETIC WAVES

Electromagnetic radiation can be defined as the propagation of energy through space by (as the name suggests) electric and magnetic fields that vary in time.

We are not going to describe varying electric fields here; instead, we intend only to describe the magnetic field components of electromagnetic radiation. This field can be thought of as a magnetic field that oscillates; that is, it rises and falls with time in a sinusoidal way. It can be generated by an antenna: For example, an oscillating electric current (an alternating current) flowing in the wire of the antenna shown in Fig. 3-4 will cause an oscillating magnetic field to travel outward from the antenna; at any point distant from the antenna the strength of the magnetic field can be measured. As we have seen, magnetic fields can induce currents as well as result from them; therefore, if another antenna were set up at this distant point, an alternating current would be induced in it by the oscillating magnetic field in which it exists (see Fig. 3-4). Under these circumstances, one antenna can be thought of as sending a signal to the other antenna.

There is another way an oscillating magnetic field can be generated. Imagine that a bar magnet is placed sufficiently near a wire so that the wire is within the magnetic field of

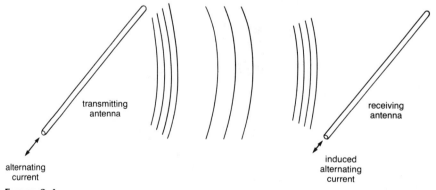

transmitting antenna

receiving antenna

alternating current

induced alternating current

FIGURE 3-4.
The transmitting antenna is a wire with an alternating current. The alternating current sets up a magnetic field around the wire, whose strength at any point oscillates as the current in the wire alternates. If a wire acting as a receiving antenna rests within the oscillating magnetic field, it will have an alternating current induced within it.

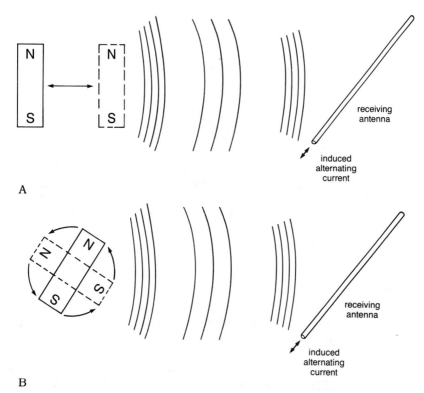

FIGURE 3-5.
Oscillating magnetic field. A. A magnet moved back and forth will create a
magnetic field, whose strength at any point rises and falls as the magnet
moves. As in Fig. 3-4, a wire acting as a receiving antenna will have an
alternating current induced within it as the magnetic lines of flux move back
and forth across it. B. A similar effect is created if the magnet revolves
(around any axis other than its north-south axis) instead of moving back
and forth.

the bar magnet (Fig. 3-5). Now imagine that the magnet is
moved back and forth in such a way that it moves first closer
to and then farther away from the wire. The wire will then
experience a surrounding magnetic field that rises and falls
in strength, which requires that magnetic lines of flux move
across the wire. This will induce an oscillating voltage (and
hence an alternating current) in the wire, and the wire will
act exactly as the receiving antenna did in Fig. 3-4. Alternatively, the magnet could be spun around an axis *other* than
the one between its north and south poles, so that a given
pole travels at first toward and then away from the receiving
antenna (see Fig. 3-5). Either type of motion of the magnet
will generate an oscillating magnetic field (which, if the fre-

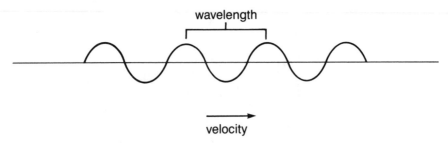

wavelength

velocity

FIGURE 3-6.
A simple representation of an oscillating magnetic field. This constitutes a radio wave that moves at the speed of light and has a particular wavelength. The *frequency* of the signal is inversely proportional to the wavelength.

quency of the oscillations is within the radio frequency band of the entire electromagnetic spectrum, is known as a radio frequency field), which can then be detected by the receiving wire.

This oscillating magnetic field may be drawn as a sinusoidal wave (Fig. 3-6). A radio frequency wave, being part of the electromagnetic spectrum, travels (at least in a vacuum) with the speed of light, and has a wavelength that is inversely proportional to its frequency. The range of possible frequencies with which energy can be thus radiated varies tremendously, from high-energy gamma rays with frequencies in the order of 10^{23} to 10^{24} Hz down to radio frequency waves with frequencies in the range of 10^4 to 10^8 Hz (a *Hertz*, abbreviated Hz, is one cycle per second). It is at the low end of this range that NMR phenomena occur. And since the energy of electromagnetic waves is proportional to the frequency, the energy of the waves is at the low end of the spectrum.

The magnetic fields of such radio frequency waves may interact in predictable ways. For example, two sets of waves may be identical in frequency and phase; these may be added to form a signal that has the same frequency but an increased amplitude, which is the sum of the amplitudes of the two individual waves. Or two waves may be of similar frequency but opposing phase; when added together, they will produce a signal of the original frequency, but diminished amplitude. Finally, two or more waves of different amplitudes and frequencies may be added together to produce a very complex wave.

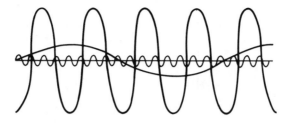

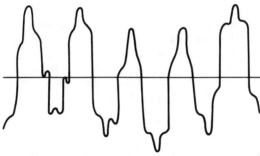

FIGURE 3-7.
Radio frequency waves of different frequencies and amplitudes. The top part of the diagram reveals three separate radio frequency waves all drawn on the same horizontal axis. If the waves are added together, the resultant single waveform will look like that in the lower part of the diagram. Fourier analysis of the lower waveform could separate it into the three original components.

Figure 3-7 shows what happens if three waves of different frequencies and amplitudes are added together. Such a complex waveform can be subjected to analysis by a process known as *Fourier transformation*; this sort of analysis might take the waveform seen on the bottom of Fig. 3-7 and determine the amplitude, or amount of energy, expressed in each of the frequencies of the waves' components (Fig. 3-8). Notice that the three peaks in Fig. 3-8 correspond to the three different frequencies and three different amplitudes of the individual signals seen on the top of Fig. 3-7.

Up until this point, we have discussed concepts that are relatively general, albeit necessary to understand MRI. From this point on, we intend to discuss some more specific issues: These are the events that actually occur within an MRI

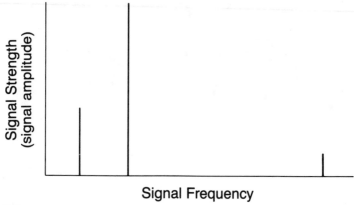

Signal Frequency

FIGURE 3-8.
If the composite radio frequency signal illustrated on the bottom of Fig. 3-7 were subjected to Fourier analysis, which could separate it into its three components and assign the correct amplitude and frequency for each component, the resulting information could be displayed this way. Comparison of this figure with that on the top of Fig. 3-7 shows that each figure describes the frequency and amplitude of the three individual signals. Information regarding the phase of the individual signals is missing in Fig. 3-8, however.

device. We intend to concentrate on the phenomena that are peculiar to the anatomy and pathology which are ultimately displayed by MRI, and that are within the control of the operator of an MRI device. The functions of an MRI device that cannot be manipulated directly by the imager are discussed relatively briefly, despite their obvious importance to the operation of the machine and their interest to scientists who develop the machines.

CHAPTER 4

Tissue Magnetization

In all NMR imaging, the body part from which an image is to be made is subjected to a relatively powerful magnetic field, which is generated by a magnet that surrounds the body.

The consequence of placing tissue in a strong magnetic field is that the tissue itself acquires a net magnetization; that is, it acts like a magnet generating a magnetic field of its own. Why this comes about, and how this tissue magnetization acts, are important to know in order to understand NMR imaging.

Any atomic nucleus whose total number of protons and neutrons is an odd number can be viewed as if it is a small magnet itself. Like any other magnet, each nucleus can be viewed as a magnetic dipole; that is, it has a north pole and a south pole. The consequence of this is that the magnetic field caused by each nucleus has a particular direction. As we discussed earlier, this field can be described by a vector. Figure 4-1 illustrates these notions: A hypothetic proton is represented as if it had a north and south magnetic pole; it generates a magnetic field around itself, which is identical to that which might be produced by a tiny bar magnet with a north and south pole. The nucleus is then depicted as a small sphere that spins around an axis and contains a charge; a spinning charge is, for all practical purposes, a current flowing in a circle, and, as we have seen, a current flowing in a circle produces a magnetic field with a particular shape. In any case, the magnetic fields of all three concepts look identical, and can be drawn as a vector, which has, like all vectors, both direction and magnitude.

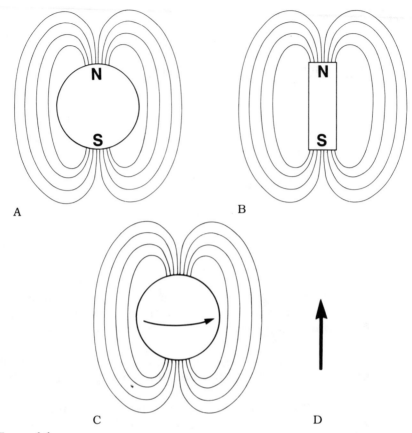

FIGURE 4-1.
A. The magnetic field produced by a hydrogen nucleus (proton), which can be viewed as if it has a north and south pole. B. The magnetic field generated by a hypothetic tiny bar magnet. C. The magnetic field generated by a charge spinning about a sphere. Note that the fields are identical. D. The fields can be represented by a vector.

When the tissue is not subjected to an externally applied magnetic field, the orientation or direction of the fields of the nuclei is random (Fig. 4-2) and varies randomly with time. But when the tissue is placed in a magnetic field, the field exerts a force on these randomly oriented nuclear magnetizations so that they tend to align themselves with the externally applied field (Fig. 4-3A). The result of this is that the net nuclear magnetization of the tissue is aligned parallel to the externally applied field (Fig. 4-3B). The tissue has now become a weak magnet.

There are several important points to understand about this tissue magnetization. First of all, if the tissue is instantly exposed to the externally applied field, it will not be-

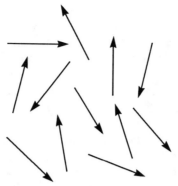

FIGURE 4-2.
Each vector represents the magnetization of an individual proton in a fluid or tissue that is not subjected to an external magnetic field. (This is an oversimplification; each vector also has a spin, and the direction of the vectors changes randomly with time.)

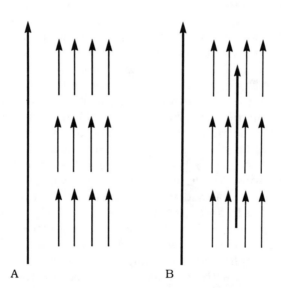

A   B

FIGURE 4-3.
A. Vectors (small arrows) of the magnetizations of individual protons in a tissue or fluid subjected to a strong magnetic field (large arrow). (This, too, is an oversimplification; each individual proton's vector has a spin, the direction only approximates that of the external field, and the direction changes with time.) B. The *net* magnetic vector of the tissue or fluid caused by the aligned protons' magnetizations (medium-length arrow). This net magnetic vector can also be viewed as if it has a spin, but despite the slight variations of directions of the protons' individual vectors, its direction remains constant.

come a magnet instantly itself; rather, its magnetization will grow at first rapidly and then more slowly, ultimately reaching a certain value (Fig. 4-4). This might be understood as a process that reflects the time necessary for the randomly moving nuclear magnetizations to become lined up with the externally applied field (Fig. 4-5). A second point is that the ultimate strength of the tissue magnetization is directly related to the strength of the externally applied field. It is also related to characteristics of the tissue itself. Different tissues in the same magnetic field may acquire different ultimate magnetizations. The degree to which a tissue acquires magnetization in response to magnetic fields to which it is exposed is called the tissue's *magnetic susceptibility.*

A third point is that by no means do all of the nuclear magnetizations align with the externally applied field (therefore, the situation depicted at the right of Fig. 4-6 is never really achieved). A more accurate way to view the situation would be to see the individual nuclear magnetizations as continuing to change their orientations constantly, but to have a tendency to spend more of their time with their magnetizations partially or completely aligned with the externally applied field. The dependence of the strength of the tissue magnetization on the strength of the externally applied field thus becomes more apparent. The stronger the externally applied field is, the harder it "tugs" on all of the nuclear magnetizations, and the more time they tend to spend aligned with the external field. (It is important not to confuse the model of classic mechanics and magnetism that we have been using with the model of quantum theory. In the latter case, each nuclear magnetization is thought of as being only directly aligned with the externally applied field or directly opposed to it. In this model, if a tissue is not subjected to an external magnetic field, the number of nuclear magnetizations oriented in one direction is the same as the number of those oriented in the other. As a magnetic field is applied, at any instant more nuclear magnetizations are aligned with the applied field than against it, with the imbalance becoming stronger as the strength of the applied field grows. But as we mentioned, for the purposes of this book, we are going to use a classic model rather than the quantum model to explain the phenomena.)

Let us get back to tissue magnetization. As we said, any nucleus with an odd number of protons and neutrons can have a magnetization and thus contribute to the net magnetization of tissue once the tissue is placed in a magnetic field. However, most NMR imaging depends on the magnetization of a particular species—the single proton that is the

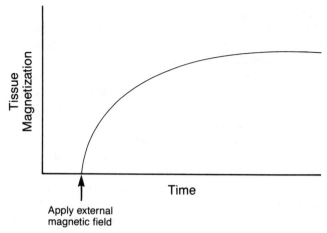

FIGURE 4-4.
Magnetization acquired by tissue when exposed to an external magnetic field. Note that the tissue magnetization grows at first rapidly, and then slowly asymptotically approaches a constant level.

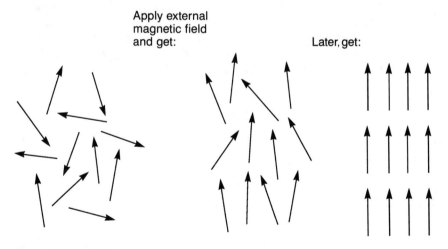

FIGURE 4-5.
Response of protons' magnetizations to application of an external field. Their alignment does not appear instantly, but requires a finite time.

nucleus of the hydrogen atom. There are several reasons for this. As we are going to see, it is the tissue's magnetization that enables it to emit the radio frequency signal from which images are made. Since there is more hydrogen than any other element in human tissue, and since hydrogen is particularly good at producing the tissue magnetization ultimately necessary to cause the tissue to emit radio frequency signal, the contribution of hydrogen to the radio frequency signal that tissue emits is particularly strong. It is possible to do NMR imaging with other nuclei, but it is more difficult than imaging with protons.

The most abundant compound containing hydrogen in tissue is water. It is often said that proton NMR imaging is the imaging of water. But hydrogen atoms are also in fat and other lipids, and these are imaged as well.

To summarize, hydrogen nuclei (protons) in tissue are abundant and act like small, moving, randomly oriented bar magnets. When tissue is exposed to a strong magnetic field from an external magnet, the nuclei tend to orient their magnetizations parallel with the field, so that the tissue itself becomes magnetized. This tissue magnetization is oriented in the same direction as the main magnetic field and grows to a strength proportional to the strength of the externally applied field, and is also proportional to each tissue's magnetic susceptibility. The magnetization of tissue is what will allow the tissue to emit radio frequency energy and permit an image to be made.

CHAPTER 5

Tissue Absorption and Emission of Radio Frequency Energy

ABSORPTION OF RADIO FREQUENCY ENERGY

Before we can go any further with this discussion, it is important to know that each nucleus not only has a characteristic of magnetization, but also has a characteristic of spin. In our simple classic model, each nucleus can be viewed as if it is a small bar magnet that spins about its north pole—south pole axis; therefore, the net magnetic vector of tissue that has been placed in a magnetic field can also be viewed as if it has a "spin." A volume of tissue can then be regarded as acting as if it is a larger bar magnet that spins around its north pole—south pole axis. This quality of spin is particularly important in the subsequent discussion.

Now let us go back to our system in which a body has been placed in a strong magnetic field and its tissue has become magnetized. Let us add to that system a radio frequency signal. This can be done simply by placing a coil of wire near the tissue and running an alternating current through it; the coil thus becomes a radio frequency transmitting antenna (Fig. 5-1).

Radio frequency signal (an oscillating magnetic field) is now applied to the tissue along with the stationary field, which has been applied by the main magnet. The oscillating magnetic field is orders of magnitude weaker than the stationary field, but it nevertheless has an effect on tissue magnetization, and the tissue magnetization responds to it.

Let us look at the magnetization vectors that are affected. Figure 5-2 demonstrates the tissue magnetization vector M,

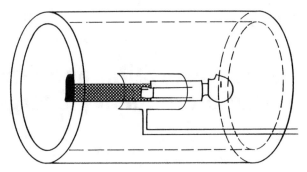

FIGURE 5-1.
The hollow cylinder representing a solenoidal magnet, whose core contains a magnetic field. A patient is seen within the field. The loop of wire around the patient functions as a radio frequency transmitting antenna.

which has been produced by the large main magnetic field into which the tissue has been placed. (Note that the vector is drawn as if it is in the Z direction. This direction is drawn as a vertical one despite the fact that in most clinical imaging magnets the direction of the main magnetic field is horizontal. This is merely a matter of convention, but it is an important one: The Z direction is virtually always drawn as a vertical direction, and tissue magnetization, which is parallel to the main magnetic field, always points in the Z direction.) Tissue magnetization in the Z direction is also known as "longitudinal" magnetization. Incidentally, we have also drawn the main external magnetic field as a vector, labeled "B_0," which is considerably stronger than the tissue magnetization and parallel to it. In fact, the main magnetic

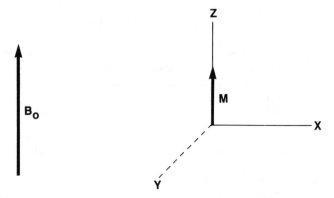

FIGURE 5-2.
The net magnetization vector (M) of a tissue has been drawn on our three-dimensional coordinate system. The tissue magnetization has been induced by the applied field B_0.

field is orders of magnitude stronger than the tissue magnetization.

The oscillating magnetic field—that is, the radio frequency field set up by the transmitting coil within the magnet—is oriented so that its vectors are always in the XY plane; it exerts a force on the tissue magnetization that is always *perpendicular* to the main magnetic field. But the force is, of course, not constant in direction, since the direction of the field oscillates or rotates. This force causes the net magnetic vector of the tissue to begin to oscillate in the XY plane.

The usual analogy to explain this phenomenon is that of a spinning toy top. Let us consider a top that is spinning on a flat surface, and suppose that its axis of spin is directly lined up with a force (the earth's gravitational force). If nothing else happens to the top, it would continue to spin and its axis of spin will not move. This is analogous to the spinning net magnetic vector of the tissue being directly aligned with the main magnetic field (the field in the Z direction). Now let us suppose that the upper end of the top is given a very brief push in a horizontal direction; it might be quickly flicked with a finger (Fig. 5-3). The top would then begin to wobble slightly; this wobbling motion is known as *precession*. It is important to note that the frequency of the spin of the top around its own axis is not the same as the frequency of the precessional motion. The frequency of the precessional motion is due to some characteristics of the top itself (including its mass) and is directly proportional to the force of gravity. If, for example, we did exactly the same top-flicking experiment on the moon, where the gravitational force is less, the corresponding precessional frequency would be less. Alternatively, if we performed it on Jupiter, where the gravitational pull is very strong, the frequency would be considerably higher than it is on Earth. In any case, the top will adopt a natural precessional frequency depending on both internal and external characteristics.

Now let us suppose that the finger flicks the top repeatedly and at a fixed interval. If the flicks occur at the same frequency as the natural precessional frequency of the top (so that each time the top is pushed in a horizontal direction, it is already moving in that direction), the angle of precession will grow greater and greater. If the frequency of flicks is *not* the same as the precessional frequency, repeated flicks will *not* cause the precessional angle to increase. This principle might be even easier to comprehend by thinking of pushing a child's swing: If the swing is pushed forward each time its natural swing frequency makes it go forward anyway, the

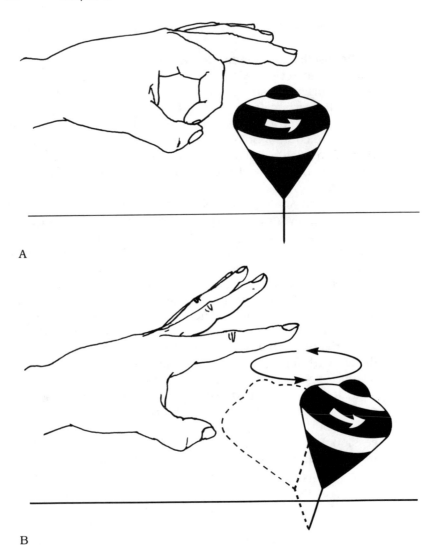

A

B

FIGURE 5-3.
A. The top spins around its long axis, which is stationary. B. The finger has flicked the top and the axis of rotation now precesses, or travels in a cone-shaped path. The precession of the axis is distinct from the spin of the top around the axis.

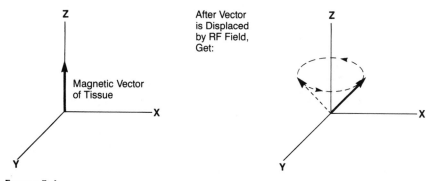

Figure 5-4.
The magnetic vector of a tissue (the vector of the field that has been applied to induce the tissue magnetization has not been drawn). After the vector has been displaced by the transient application of a radio frequency (RF) field, the vector precesses around the Z axis.

swing will move through a wider and wider angle. Most other patterns of pushes on the swing will push against the natural motion of the swing as often as it pushes with the motion, and the net amplitude of the swing's motion will not increase.

To get back to our magnetized tissue, the net magnetic vector of the tissue is acted on by the static magnetic field (corresponding to the pull of gravity in the top model) and also by the rotating magnetic field (corresponding to the repetitive horizontal flicks in the top model) (Fig. 5-4). As long as the frequency of the rotating magnetic field (which is, of course, the frequency of the radio frequency signal) is identical to the precessional frequency of the vector, the angle through which the vector precesses will continue to increase more and more. Next comes an important point: *The precessional frequency of the tissue's net magnetic vector is directly proportional to the strength of the static magnetic field* (remember the dependence of the top's precessional frequency on gravity?). Therefore, energy can be transferred from the radio frequency wave to the tissue magnetization *if* the frequency of the radio frequency signal is just right. The longer this signal is applied, the greater is the change in the angle of precession. The angle of precession can also be affected by the strength of the radio frequency signal; a strong signal of the correct frequency can cause the precession angle to change faster than a weak signal can. A signal exactly strong enough and applied for a requisite period of time to increase the precessional angle by 90 degrees is called a 90-degree pulse (Fig. 5-5).

It is important to remember that the net magnetic vector

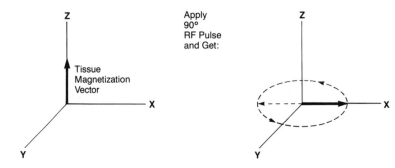

The tissue magnetization vector has been caused to precess by the application of a longer (or stronger) radio frequency (RF) pulse than that depicted in Fig. 5-4. The vector now precesses at an angle of 90 degrees from its original position (that is, at 90 degrees from the Z axis).

of the tissue is made up of all of the components contributed by the individual magnetizations of the protons. Each of their precessional frequencies also directly depends on the strength of the main magnetic field and, as long as the field is exactly the same for all protons, they will continue to precess in phase with each other (which, of course, is necessary if there is to be a precessing net magnetic vector at all). The net magnetic vector is always the sum of the vectors of the individual protons.

The relationship between the strength of the main magnetic field and the precessional frequency of the magnetic vectors is known as the Larmor relationship. Mathematically, it is stated as follows:

$$f = \frac{\gamma B}{2\pi}$$

where f is the frequency of precession, B is the strength of the net magnetic field, and γ is the magnetogyric (or gyromagnetic) ratio. The *magnetogyric ratio* is a constant for each nucleus. The magnetogyric ratio for protons is such that the precessional frequency for the protons' magnetization is about 42 MHz for a magnetic field of 1 Tesla.

Although the formula itself is not essential to remember, it is important to keep in mind that the frequency of the absorbed radio frequency energy is directly proportional to the strength of the static magnetic field. Incidentally, one of the reasons it is important to have a homogeneous magnetic field should now be apparent: If the main field is different in a small region from what it is thought to be, the effect of the radio frequency pulses on the tissue magnetization will be altered.

To summarize, the tissue within the static magnetic field can also be exposed to a radio frequency signal, which consists of a magnetic field whose direction oscillates within the XY plane. If the frequency of oscillation is exactly the same as the precessional frequency of the tissue's magnetic vector, the vector can be made to move out of alignment with the main magnetic field and to precess around the Z axis. The longer the radio frequency field is applied and the stronger it is, the greater will be the resulting angle of precession. The direct linear relationship between the frequency of precession and the strength of the main magnetic field is known as the Larmor relationship.

EMISSION OF SIGNAL

Next we need to consider the consequences of a precessing tissue magnetization. Let us suppose that the tissue's net magnetization is precessing at an angle of 90 degrees from the Z direction; that is, it is precessing exactly within the XY plane. The same thing happens as would happen if an actual magnet were being spun around and around within the XY plane (recall Fig. 3-5). Since the shape of the magnetic field generated by a magnet is determined by, among other things, the position of its north and south poles, if these poles spin around in a plane, the strength of the magnetic field within the plane will oscillate with the same frequency as the precession of the magnetic dipole. Now remember that the radio frequency signal is an oscillating magnetic field; it follows that *a precessing tissue magnetic vector will cause a radio frequency signal to be emitted* (Fig. 5-6). This signal can be detected by a conducting wire. Since such a wire will have a current induced in it if it is subjected to a changing field, and since the strength of the field at any point is oscillating because the tissue magnetization is precessing, the wire will have an alternating current induced in it and become a receiving antenna. In short, a precessing tissue magnetic vector will cause a radio frequency signal to be generated, which in turn can be detected by using an antenna that will have an alternating current induced within it.

A few points need emphasizing. That part of the tissue magnetization which is in the XY plane moves in a circle. Since magnetization in the XY plane is never stationary, but

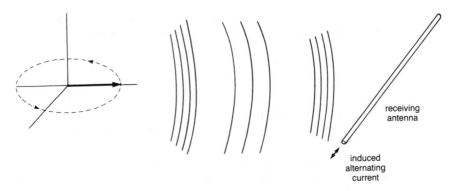

receiving antenna

induced alternating current

FIGURE 5-6.
Magnetization precessing in a transverse plane causes an oscillating magnetic field in the vicinity of the precessing magnetization. This oscillating field can induce an alternating voltage in a wire that acts as a receiving antenna within the field.

always precesses around the Z axis, it is usually not necessary to speak of magnetization in the X direction or magnetization in the Y direction; the magnetization is never stationary in either of these directions. Therefore, we only speak of magnetization rotating in the XY plane. This plane is also known as the *transverse plane*, and magnetization in it is also known as *transverse magnetization*.

Magnetization in the transverse plane causes a radio frequency signal to be emitted. The frequency of the signal will, of course, be the same as the frequency of precession, which, in turn, will be directly proportional to the strength of the magnetic field according to the Larmor relationship. If the strength of the static magnetic field should change between the time a radio frequency pulse is applied and the time the tissue emits radio frequency signals of its own, the Larmor relationship still holds: The frequency of the signal that will be absorbed during the radio frequency pulse will be directly proportional to the magnetic field strength *at that time*, and the frequency of the radio frequency signal that is subsequently emitted will be directly proportional to the strength of the field that exists *when the signal is being emitted*.

Finally, as might be imagined, the strength, or amplitude, of the emitted signal is directly proportional to the strength of the magnetization in the XY plane. If there is no magnetization in the XY plane, no signal will be emitted.

It is worth remembering that any magnetization in the Z direction, since it does not oscillate, will not emit a signal; the signal that is being emitted is in no way affected by the size of any simultaneous magnetization in the Z direction.

CHAPTER 6

Image Contrast, Relaxation Processes, and Pulse Sequences

So far, we have described the process by which tissue can be made to emit a radio frequency signal: It is subjected to a strong static magnetic field and to a pulse (or pulses) of radio frequency energy, which in turn gives the tissue a magnetization that rotates in the XY plane and causes a radio frequency signal to be emitted. We also mentioned that the emitted signal is detected by an antenna and ultimately is used as the basic information from which to generate an image. Two major topics now need to be approached: the processes by which *spatial information* is acquired and displayed in the image—that is, the tricks an MRI device uses to figure out the exact location in the body from which each portion of the emitted radio frequency signal originates, which is of course necessary to create an image; and how *contrast information* is determined—that is, how each pixel in the image is determined to be white, black, or a shade of gray. We deal with the latter in this chapter.

In most clinical MR images, the gray scale finally depends on one thing, the strength of the radio frequency signal that is emitted by each voxel. A *voxel* is that volume of tissue represented by a single pixel on the image. The stronger the signal being emitted from a voxel is, the brighter the image will be (Fig. 6-1). This is directly comparable to an x-ray computed tomograph, in which the brightness of each region of the image is directly proportional to the x-ray attenuation of the corresponding piece of tissue.

The intensity of the signal emitted from each voxel of tissue is, as we have seen, proportional to the strength of the transverse magnetization of that portion of tissue. As one

43

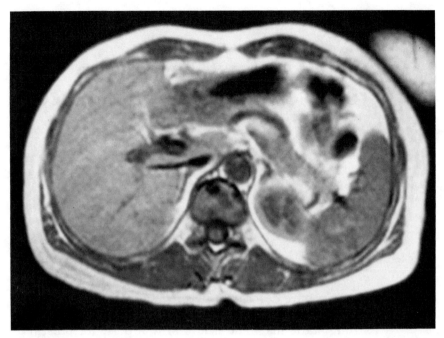

FIGURE 6-1.
MR image. As with all MR images, the brightness of any region in the image is proportional to the strength of the radio frequency signal that is emitted from the corresponding tissue. In this case, subcutaneous fat emits a particularly strong signal; liver, spleen, and muscle emit intermediate signal strengths; and air in the stomach emits negligible signal. The emitted signal from each tissue is proportional to that tissue's transverse magnetization. Fat has a strong transverse magnetization; the liver, spleen, and muscle have intermediate strength; and air has negligible magnetization.

might imagine, since the radio frequency signal emitted is produced by the rotating magnetization in the tissue, the larger the transverse magnetization is, the stronger the radio frequency signal will be. So in the end, what determines contrast in MRI is the *strength of the transverse magnetization* in the various parts of the tissue imaged (see Fig. 6-1).

The transverse magnetization, in turn, is affected by a number of things, of which we intend to discuss only the four most important.

These are:

1. The mobile proton density (or spin density).
2. T1 (or spin-lattice or longitudinal) relaxation.
3. T2 (or spin-spin or transverse) relaxation.
4. Tissue motion, of which blood flow is the most important example.

We recognize that the first three of these four items may be entirely unfamiliar to you; we will define these as we go along. Blood flow will be discussed in Chapter 9.

MOBILE PROTON DENSITY

Recall that hydrogen nuclei (individual protons) are the atomic species that creates the tissue magnetization we are imaging, and that these nuclei can change the orientation of their magnetizations when a static magnetic field is applied to them and when a rotating magnetic field (a radio frequency signal) is applied as well. But some protons are in a state in which the transverse magnetizations produce a net tissue transverse magnetization that is extremely short-lived (that is, it has a very short T2, a phenomenon we have not discussed yet but which we will deal with later on) and do not generate sufficient radio frequency signal to contribute to the image: These tissues are said to have a low mobile proton density (although their overall proton density may not differ much from other tissues). Cortical bone and certain fibrous tissues have low mobile proton densities, and hence always look very dark or black on an MR image (Fig. 6-2). Of course, where there are very few protons, there

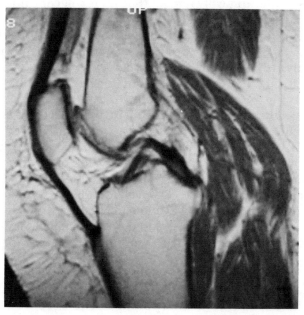

FIGURE 6-2.
MR image of the knee. Cortical bone, the quadriceps and patellar tendons, and the cruciate ligaments appear quite dark because they have low mobile proton density and can emit little signal.

can be very little net magnetization and hence little signal can be emitted; parts of the anatomy that are made up primarily of air (such as bubbles within the gastrointestinal tract, and the airways, peripheral lung tissue, and aerated sinuses of the respiratory system) also always look black and are also said to have a low proton density (see Fig. 6-1). In tissues in which there is a significant amount of mobile protons (essentially, every other tissue in the body), the intensity of the signal and hence the brightness of the tissues as they appear on the images follow more complex rules. These we will discuss shortly.

RELAXATION PROCESSES

T1 Relaxation

To begin a discussion of tissue relaxation, let us consider some tissue—a cubic centimeter of liver, for example—resting in a static magnetic field. As we have seen, this tissue will have acquired a magnetization of its own, which will be in the same direction as that of the applied static field. It has a longitudinal magnetization and will have no transverse magnetization. If we observe this tissue over a length of time, nothing will change; that is, it will continue to have a longitudinal magnetization of a constant strength.

But now let us imagine what would occur the instant the tissue is placed in the field. If it were moved into the field extremely suddenly, or if the field were turned on extremely suddenly, there would be an instant in which the tissue existed in the field but had not yet acquired any longitudinal magnetization. (This experiment is not actually performed during MRI, but it is useful as a simplified hypothetic situation.) That tissue magnetization would take a finite time to appear; it would grow from a value of zero to approach asymptotically its final strength (see Figs. 4-5 and 4-6). Remember that this process involves individual proton magnetizations oriented in random directions and moving randomly until they are exposed to the main magnetic field, after which they begin to line up in the same direction as the field.

This process—aligning the individual protons with the subsequent growth of the tissues' net magnetization—is a *relaxation process*. It may seem odd at first that we describe the acquisition of magnetization by tissue as relaxation; it might seem to make more sense that magnetic relaxation would describe the loss of magnetization. However, if a tissue in a strong magnetic field has its own magnetization parallel to that magnetic field, it is in a relatively low-energy state with regard to the field. On the other hand, if it had a magnetization pointing in a direction other than that of the main field (or, for that matter, if it were in a state of having no magnetization at all), the tissue magnetization might be seen to be at a relatively high-energy state with respect to the main magnetic field; that is, it is opposed to that main field in some way. So when the tissues' magnetization ultimately aligns itself *with* the field, it is said to have relaxed. An intuitive way to imagine this might be to think of a bird perched on a telephone wire. As long as the bird is upright, his orientation is directly opposed to the pull of gravity. If he were to lose his balance and turn upside down, but continued to hold on to the wire with his feet, his body axis is now aligned *with* the gravitational field and he could be said to have undergone relaxation with respect to the gravitational field. In short, when a tissue's magnetization has grown to its maximum value in the same direction as the applied static field, it is said to have undergone a kind of relaxation. This particular kind of relaxation is known as *longitudinal relaxation, T1 relaxation,* or *spin-lattice relaxation.*

This sort of relaxation is very important in MRI; it is one of the major factors that control tissue contrast. There are several things that must be understood about it.

First of all, T1 relaxation is an exponential process. That is, it does not begin at some instant and become suddenly complete at another instant. Instead, longitudinal magnetization grows at a rate such that in a given period of time, a given *fraction* of the remaining relaxation—that is, a given fraction of the remaining magnetization to be acquired— takes place. The convention is to state that the *relaxation time* of a particular tissue or substance is the time required for approximately 63 percent of the remaining relaxation to take place. So, as we have said, relaxation approaches its maximum value asymptotically. To be absolutely rigid about it, it is never entirely complete, but in practical terms, relaxation is essentially complete within four or five relaxation times from the beginning of the process (see Fig. 4-5).

The other important thing about relaxation is that soft tissues in the body have decidedly different relaxation times. In aqueous tissues, relaxation appears to be a function (among other things) of the concentration of proteins and other macromolecules within the water of the tissue. These vary from normal tissue to normal tissue, so that liver, kidney, spleen, brain gray matter, and muscle all tend to differ in their T1 values. Tissues that contain a high proportion of lipid, such as fat and the white matter of the brain, have relatively fast (or short) T1 times. What is perhaps more important is that in tissues that are inflamed or edematous or have undergone malignant transformation, the amount of free water increases (that is, the concentration of macromolecules decreases), so that the T1 relaxation time of tissues that have been altered in these ways increases. Later we will see how these differences in T1 relaxation time can be translated into differences in image intensity, and hence permit detection of pathology.

T1 values tend to increase as the strength of the magnetic field increases. The relative differences among the T1 values of different tissues decrease, however, as field strength increases.

To summarize, (1) T1 relaxation is the process by which the magnetization of a tissue approaches the constant magnetization induced by a constant applied magnetic field; (2) longitudinal (or T1) relaxation specifically refers to the growth of longitudinal magnetization; (3) the T1 relaxation time is defined as the time required for approximately 63 percent of the remaining longitudinal magnetization to appear; (4) tissues differ in their T1 values; and (5) in general, the more "watery" the tissue is, the longer its T1 relaxation time will be. The T1 relaxation times for substances encountered in clinical MRI practice using common field strengths ranged from about 2,000 milliseconds for urine to a value of somewhere between 100 and 200 milliseconds for fat.

T2 Relaxation

Now that we have defined T1 relaxation as a growth of tissue magnetization parallel to the direction of the main magnetic field, the other kind of relaxation that we must consider is *T2* (or *transverse*, or *spin-spin*) *relaxation.*

To understand this, let us imagine a piece of tissue—our cubic centimeter of liver again—in a strong magnetic field. Let us suppose that it has just been exposed to a 90-degree pulse of radio frequency energy so that its net magnetization vector is now precessing in a plane perpendicular to the main magnetic field; that is, it is precessing in the plane defined by the X and Y axes of our usual three-dimensional coordinate system or, to put it in yet another way, it is precessing in the *transverse* plane. It is, of course, emitting a radio frequency signal. Figure 6-3 shows what happens to the individual magnetization of six protons in the tissue. At

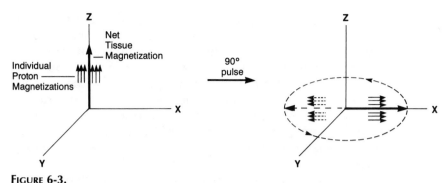

FIGURE 6-3.
The vectors of individual proton magnetizations (small arrows) are parallel, in response to an applied magnetic field. Their sum is the larger vector, which represents the net tissue magnetization. After a 90-degree radio frequency pulse, the individual proton magnetizations initially remain parallel; they and their resultant net tissue magnetization precess at an angle of 90 degrees to the Z axis.

first, their magnetizations add up to a net tissue magnetization oriented in the Z direction. After a 90-degree pulse, the individual proton magnetizations precess in the transverse plane, and thus produce a net tissue magnetization precessing in the transverse plane.

Looking at Fig. 6-3, we can see that the net magnetization of the tissue is made up of the individual magnetization vectors of the individual protons. These are aligned with each other, which is necessary if they are going to generate a net vector, and precess at the same rate so that they continue to be aligned. Now we must remember what controls the speed, or the frequency, with which the individual protons precess. The Larmor relationship, which we described before, requires that the protons precess at a frequency that is directly proportional to the strength of the main magnetic field. For them to continue to precess at identical values, the magnetic field would have to be an absolutely uniform one; that is, as one moves from place to place within it, one finds that it has exactly the same strength throughout. (This, as we have stated, is impossible. No one can build a magnet that has an absolutely uniform field. But for the purposes of this part of the discussion, let us assume that the field is uniform.) One might think, then, that protons anywhere within the imaged tissue will precess at the same rate, so that they will stay aligned forever. But in fact this does *not* happen. In tissue, there are multiple moving charged particles, including electrons and nuclear particles, and moving charged particles create magnetic fields of their own. As the precessing protons move around within very small regions of the tissue, they approach or move away from the other moving charged particles in the tissue, and therefore experience changing magnetic fields. The changes in the field strength that the particles experience are very small compared with the strength of the overall field, but the changes are still real and important. The changes are also random; that is, the exact frequency of the variations in magnetic field strength and the amplitude of these variations are, in the experience of any particular precessing proton, totally unpredictable.

One can imagine what might happen as a result of all this. If there are random variations in the magnetic field that the

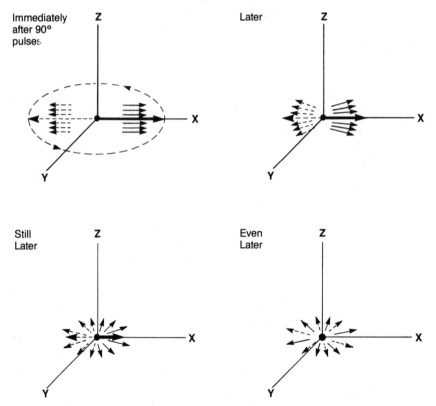

FIGURE 6-4.
Individual proton magnetizations and the net magnetization precess in the XY plane, as in Fig. 6-3, immediately after a 90-degree pulse. Later, the individual magnetizations begin to diverge somewhat, due to their random variations in precessional speed, or frequency. As they diverge, their net magnetization (the thickest arrow) shrinks. Still later, they diverge even more, and their net magnetization has diminished further. When the positions of the individual magnetic vectors have become evenly distributed in the XY (transverse) plane, their net vector has shrunk to zero.

precessing protons experience, there will also be random variations in the speed, or frequency, of their precession. Therefore, the protons will tend to fall out of alignment with each other: Even if they were perfectly aligned when they began to precess (that is, at the end of the 90-degree radio frequency pulse that started them precessing in the first place), they will ultimately become less and less aligned with each other. And what follows from this is that the *net* transverse magnetic vector of the tissue, which is the sum of the transverse magnetizations of the individual protons, will decrease (Fig. 6-4). Since the amplitude of the radio frequency signal emitted by the tissue is directly proportional to the strength of the net magnetic vector in the transverse plane, the strength of this emitted signal will also decrease (Fig. 6-5). The process by which the net magnetic vector in the transverse plane decreases is known as *transverse* (or *T2*, or *spin-spin*) *relaxation*.

T2 relaxation, like T1 relaxation, is an exponential process; the strength of the magnetization in the transverse plane approaches zero asymptotically. The same sort of terminology applied to T1 relaxation also applies to T2 relaxation. The *T2 relaxation time* is the time in which 63 percent of the remaining relaxation takes place. And although

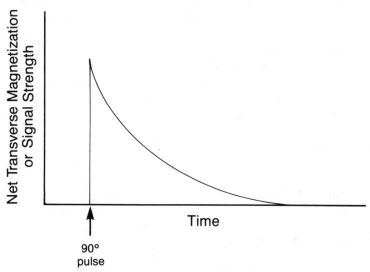

FIGURE 6-5.
The diminution of the net tissue's transverse magnetization as a function of time. It recaps the diminution of the net magnetization as shown in Fig. 6-4, and assumes a perfectly homogeneous magnetic field. The declining curve represents T2 relaxation.

theoretically T2 relaxation is never entirely complete, since it involves an asymptotic approach to a value of zero, it is, for all practical purposes, complete within four or five relaxation times of the beginning.

As with T1 relaxation, the various soft tissues of the body have different T2 relaxation times. These are, in general, much shorter than T1 relaxation times; they tend to be measured in tens of milliseconds, whereas T1 relaxation times are measured in hundreds of milliseconds. As with T1 relaxation times, T2 relaxation times elongate as tissues become more "watery"; inflamed, edematous, and malignant tissues tend to have prolonged T2 relaxation times. Fat and other lipids, however, have longer T2 relaxation times than some other soft tissues.

T2* Relaxation

Remember that for this discussion we have assumed that the main magnetic field is absolutely homogeneous. In fact, it is not; any field generated by a magnet that exists in the real world is inhomogeneous. And even though the inhomogeneities may be unchanging with time, they are relatively large, so that one portion of tissue rests in a field that is considerably stronger than the field that contains another portion. The speed of precession of the protons in the high-magnetic-field regions will, of course, be higher than the speed of precession of the protons in the low-magnetic-field region. This effect also makes the alignment of the individual protons' magnetic vectors decrease with time. In fact, the effect of this applied magnetic field inhomogeneity is usually much greater than the effect of the inhomogeneity caused by the small magnetic field variations of the tissue itself, so that the loss of net transverse magnetization occurs much more rapidly than it would if the loss were only due to the effects of the tissue. Of course, the loss of net magnetization due to the inhomogeneity of the magnetic field causes a rapid decrease in strength of emitted signal as well; Fig. 6-6 depicts the difference between the rapid diminution, or decay, of the emitted signal seen in a real situation, as opposed to what it would be if the applied magnetic field could be made absolutely homogeneous.

Therefore, the real decay of the strength of the emitted signal looks something like that seen in Fig. 6-6. This pattern of a rapidly decaying signal following a 90-degree pulse is known as the free induction decay (FID) curve. The rate of the signal's decay is, of course, much faster than that of

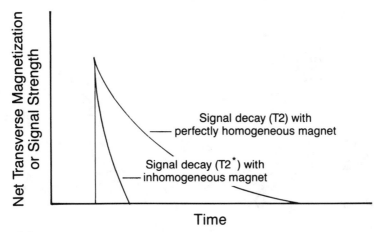

FIGURE 6-6.
The upper curve (seen also in Fig. 6-5) represents what happens in a homogeneous field after a 90-degree pulse. With an inhomogeneous magnetic field, the net transverse magnetization decays much faster. The lower curve represents the amplitude of the signal emitted by the tissue, whose decay is called T2* relaxation.

the tissue's T2 and is known as *T2**. (T2* is pronounced "Tee two star," not "Tee two asterisk.")

To view T2 relaxation in terms of a commonly used analogy, let us imagine a circular racetrack on which a foot race is to be run. Suppose that four racers of approximately equal capability begin at a starting line and run in the same direction when a gun is fired (this corresponds to the individual magnetizations of the precessing nuclei beginning to precess completely in phase at the end of a 90-degree pulse). Assume that none of these runners can maintain a constant speed, but instead each runs at a varying speed and that the speed variations of each runner are random; that is, they speed up and slow down at no particular frequency and with no particular maximum or minimum speed. With time, the runners will no longer be abreast, but will be scattered along the track in a random distribution (Fig. 6-7).

Now let us suppose that a giant hand could reach down, pluck each runner off the track, and set him down on the track again at a spot on the track opposite from where he had been along the long axis of the track (see Fig. 6-7). If this were done instantly to all runners, and the runners continued to run in the same direction and at their randomly varying speeds, not much would happen; they would continue to get more and more scattered along the track, and would never (except perhaps by some remote chance) find themselves running abreast again.

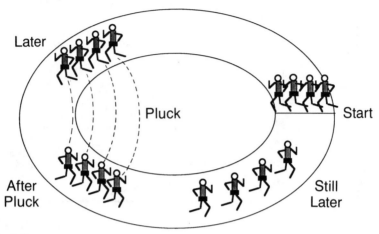

FIGURE 6-7.

Four runners on a circular track. They have approximately equal average speeds, but the speed of each varies randomly with time. Some time after the start, they are plucked from the surface of the track and placed down on the track again and continue to run in the same direction (as they are lifted from the track and replaced on it, their position is reversed; that is, the runner who was leading prior to being lifted becomes last, and the last runner becomes first). Since their speeds vary randomly, they continue to get farther apart (since the speeds vary up and down, the order of the runners in the last position may not be the same as that immediately after the pluck).

Now let us consider another variation. Instead of having the runners be of approximately the same speed but with individual random variations, we will now make our four runners intrinsically very different. The fastest will be an Olympic-class runner at the peak of training; the next fastest, a very good amateur athlete; the third, a weekend runner; and last, an elderly overweight grandmother with heart disease and bunions. Each will (let us say) continue to have momentary random variations in speed, but their overall speed differences will be much greater. The rate with which they will spread out over the track after they have started together will be very great; the Olympic runner will be shortly out of sight of the grandmother (Fig. 6-8).

Now let us do our trick of having the giant hand suddenly pluck the runners from the track and place them down on the other side of the track's axis. If the runners continue to run in the same direction, after this maneuver the fastest runner will suddenly be the farthest behind of the group and the slow grandmother will be at the head of the pack (see Fig. 6-8). Then as the Olympic runner continues to run fast and the grandmother slowly, the fast (but behind) runners

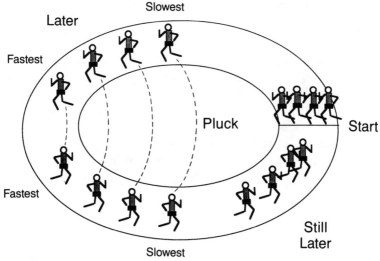

FIGURE 6-8.
Four runners on a circular track. These runners also have random intrinsic variations in speed, but, in addition, the average speed of some is greater than the average speed of others. After they have been plucked from the track and replaced on it, the slowest runners are in front of the fastest. Still later, the fastest have started to catch up with the slowest, and they are bunched closer together. The random variations in speed prevent them from ever being aligned perfectly any time after the start.

will catch up with the slow (but ahead) runners and they will shortly bunch up again on the track (see Fig. 6-8). Since they all have individual random variations in speed, they will never *exactly* be running abreast, but there will be a moment in which they are nearly at the same spot on the track. Of course, what will happen then is that the Olympic runner who is the fastest and the grandmother, the slowest, will begin to spread out along the track again, ultimately to be separated from each other by large distances.

The analogy between these runners and between T2 relaxation and T2* relaxation should now be evident. The variations in precessional speed of the protons correspond to the variations in running speed of the runners. The random small variations in the runners' speed are the same as the variations that constitute the T2 relaxation, whereas the constant large differences in runners' speed (the Olympic athlete versus the grandmother) correspond to the constant large differences among protons caused by the inhomogeneity of the applied magnetic field.

PULSE SEQUENCES

Spin Echo

But what, in an NMR experiment, might constitute the maneuver comparable to plucking the runners off one part of the track and setting them down on another? In the NMR situation, this "trick" corresponds to a 180-degree radio frequency pulse.

To look at this more closely, look at Fig. 6-9. A 90-degree pulse rotates the net magnetic vector from a stationary position in the Z direction around the Y axis into the XY plane,

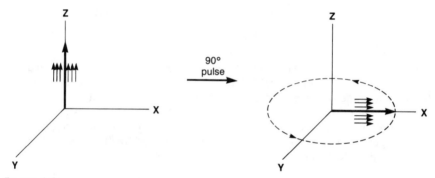

FIGURE 6-9.
Individual proton magnetizations and net tissue magnetization before and after a 90-degree pulse. These phenomena are the same as those depicted in Fig. 6-3.

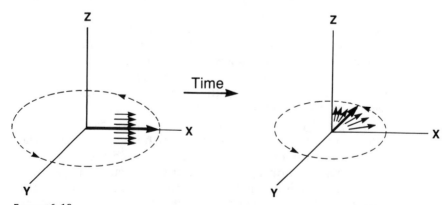

FIGURE 6-10.
Dephasing of tissue magnetization. The different positions of the individual magnetizations have been caused by random variations in speed *and* the constant differences in speeds caused by the spatial inhomogeneity of the magnetic field. The added effects constitute T2* relaxation.

where it begins to precess (like the runners) around and around in the transverse plane. After a certain period of time, the protons become out of alignment with each other (Fig. 6-10). Now let us apply a 180-degree pulse. As the 90-degree pulse rotated the magnetic vectors around the Y axis, the 180-degree pulse will do so as well (Fig. 6-11). Each proton will wind up back in the XY (or transverse) plane again, but after the 180-degree pulse, the faster protons will be behind and the slower ones ahead. As with the runners, the faster ones will then catch up with the slower ones and the protons will tend to rephase. As they do so, the net magnetic vector will increase (Fig. 6-12) and the emitted signal will grow stronger. However, as with the runners, the T2 variation in the proton precessional speed is *random*; that is, it cannot be rephased by a 180-degree pulse or any other trick. As a result, the rephasing will never be quite complete; dephasing due to the true T2 can never be recaptured.

What does this mean in terms of emitted signal? T2* will cause a rapid decay of the signal after the initial 90-degree pulse. If this is followed by a 180-degree pulse, the rephasing

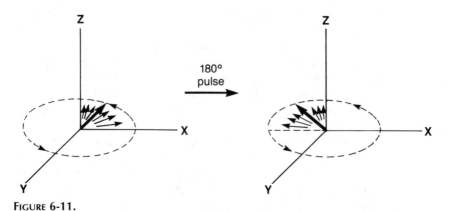

FIGURE 6-11.
The 180-degree pulse has rotated each individual vector, and the net vector, around the Y axis. The faster precessing magnetizations are now behind the slower precessing ones.

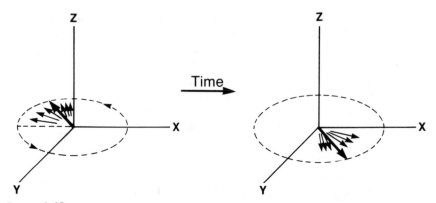

FIGURE 6-12.
After the 180-degree pulse, the faster magnetizations tend to catch up with the slower magnetizations, so that the *net* magnetization grows.

protons will cause the magnetization to increase and the signal will then regrow; once it has reached a maximum, however, the same processes that caused the initial T2* dephasing will continue, and the signal will decay. This growth and decay of a signal is known as a *spin echo*. The peak of the spin echo will never be quite as high as the peak at the beginning of the FID curve; it will be diminished by exactly the amount of true T2 relaxation that has taken place (Fig. 6-13). The time from the 90-degree pulse to the receipt of the spin echo is called *TE* (*echo time*). In the situation we have described, in which just one echo is produced, TE will be exactly twice as long as the time from the 90-degree pulse to the 180-degree pulse.

What would happen if we added another 180-degree pulse to this sequence, so that the entire pattern of applied radio frequency pulses was 90 degrees, 180 degrees, and 180 degrees? The second 180-degree pulse would reverse the positions of the individual protons' magnetizations again. That is, the fast ones would be put behind and the slow ones in front. The fast ones would then catch up with the slow ones again and all of the protons' magnetizations would rephase again. Then the emitted signal would grow again and, after the peak of the rephasing magnetization and signal has been reached, dephasing would occur with a drop in magnetization and a drop in signal. In short, a second spin echo would be emitted (Fig. 6-14). But the peak amplitude of the

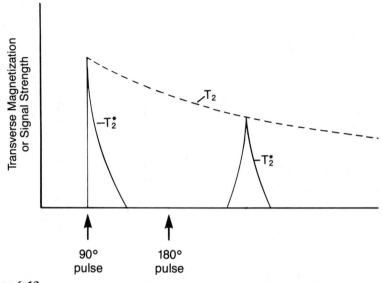

FIGURE 6-13.
Transverse magnetization with a 90-degree pulse–180-degree pulse sequence. After the 90-degree pulse, there is a rapid dephasing of transverse
magnetization (T2*). The 180-degree pulse causes a rephasing (see Fig. 6-12)
which is immediately followed by a dephasing; this rephasing and dephasing
cause a rise and fall of emitted signal, called a spin echo. The dotted line
describes T2 relaxation; that is, the decay of tissue magnetization or signal
strength that would have been seen if the process had occurred in a perfectly
homogeneous magnetic field.

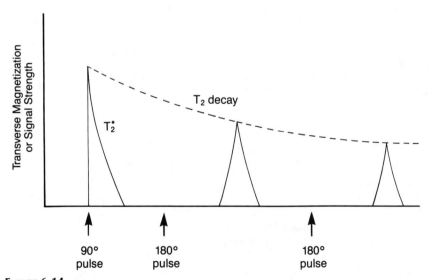

FIGURE 6-14.
A second 180-degree pulse producing a second spin echo. The apex of each
spin echo reaches the level described by the pure T2 decay curve.

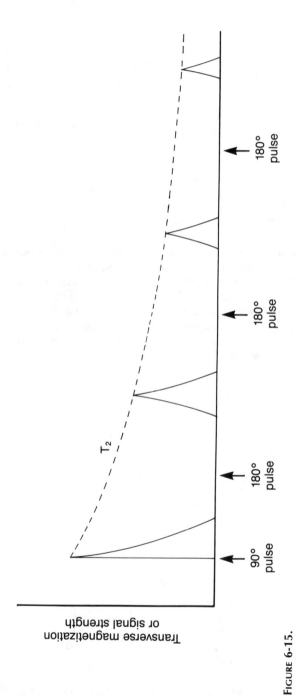

FIGURE 6-15.

Three 180-degree pulses and three spin echoes. For each spin echo, the time that elapses between the 90-degree pulse and the echo itself is known as TE (time to echo).

magnetization (and the signal) of the second spin echo would be even lower than that of the first. This is because the *random* dephasing caused by true tissue T2 relaxation processes would have been continuing the whole time and, although the nonrandom dephasing (that caused by the local fixed variations in magnetic field of the main magnet) can be rephased, the T2 dephasing caused by the tissue itself cannot.

As one might imagine, a whole series of 180-degree pulses can be applied, each of which will be followed by a spin echo (Fig. 6-15). The peak amplitude of each spin echo will be less than that of the preceding one, and a line connecting the peaks of the spin echos will itself be a decay curve that describes the rate of T2 relaxation of the tissue. This line is what we would have seen if we had given a single 90-degree pulse to a tissue in a perfectly homogeneous magnetic field. These multiple spin echoes, then, are a way of getting around the effect of the magnetic field inhomogeneity and measuring the true T2 of the tissue.

Echo Time

Remember that the emitted radio frequency signal of each spin echo can be picked up by an antenna in the MRI device (Figs. I-1 and 5-1). This antenna may be the same one that transmitted the 90-degree and 180-degree radio frequency pulse sequences in the first place (these antennae tend to be loops of wire that are arranged around the patient's periphery) or they may be separate coils of wire (a surface coil, for example, is such a separate coil). Now let us suppose that this recorded signal is used to create an image.

Let us compare two tissues with different T2 values. If we merely subjected each one to the same 90-degree pulse, each would emit an FID curve (Fig. 6-16). These curves might look nearly the same since the great portion of their decay is caused by applied magnetic field inhomogeneities, which are essentially the same in both tissues. But if we do a spin-echo experiment—that is, we apply the same 90-degree and 180-degree pulse to each of the two tissues—then a difference will become apparent. Each tissue will emit a spin echo after the 180-degree pulse, but the tissue with the shorter T2 (the one in which intrinsic T2 relaxation happens more rapidly) will emit a spin echo whose peak amplitude is considerably lower than the amplitude of the spin echo from the other tissue.

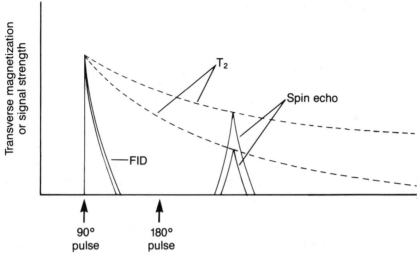

FIGURE 6-16.
The T2 curves of two tissues with different T2 values, shown by the two dotted lines. If each is subjected to a 90-degree pulse and 180-degree pulse, the amplitudes of the spin echoes that appear from each tissue will be different.

Now let us vary the time between the 90-degree and 180-degree pulses. If the pulses are very close together (Fig. 6-17), the time that elapses between the 90-degree pulse and the receipt of the spin echo will be very short. Neither tissue will have undergone much true T2 relaxation, so that the spin echo from each will be quite strong and will differ from the other very little. At the other extreme, suppose that the time between the 90-degree and 180-degree pulses is very long, each tissue will have undergone essentially *complete* T2 relaxation, so that there will be little, if any, rephasing at all. The spin echoes will be so small as to be undetectable; again, the tissues will be hard to distinguish from each other. Now let us use some intermediate value for the time between the 90-degree and 180-degree pulses (see Fig. 6-16). Here, the spin-echo signals will be easily detectable, but the tissue with the fast (or short) T2 will have undergone more random dephasing and will have a much smaller spin-echo amplitude; the tissues could be easily distinguishable, then, from the amplitude of their spin echoes.

Effect on the Image

Now let us get back to making an image. If the image is made from the emitted signal of the spin echo, and the TE

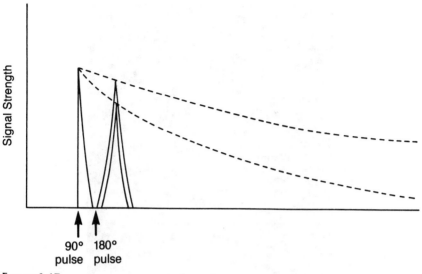

FIGURE 6-17.
If the same two tissues as in Fig. 6-16 are subjected to a 90-degree pulse and a 180-degree pulse with a short TE, the amplitudes of the two spin echoes are not greatly different.

is chosen correctly, the tissues will look quite different. The tissue with the long T2 will have a strong spin-echo signal and will look bright on the image, whereas the tissue with the fast (or short) T2 will have a weak spin-echo signal and will appear dark. Thus, an image made using a pulse sequence that produces a spin echo and with an appropriately long TE can be used whenever one wants tissues to look different from each other based on their different T2 values. Figure 6-18 is such an image; this is called a *T2-weighted* image. It reveals characteristics of all standard T2-weighted images: *Structures with relatively long T2 values appear brighter than structures with shorter T2 values.*

Incidentally, there are two other reasons to use the spin-echo sequences when performing NMR imaging. Remember that both the applied 90-degree and a 180-degree pulse sequences and the emitted signals are radio frequency signals. But the applied pulses are many orders of magnitude stronger than the received signals; Fig. 6-19 depicts a more realistic way of representing the situation. To record the entirety of the FID curve is difficult: If the receiving apparatus is set to record the FID curve right at its beginning, it is impossible to prevent the very end of the 90-degree pulse from "spilling over" into it and swamping the signal. But if

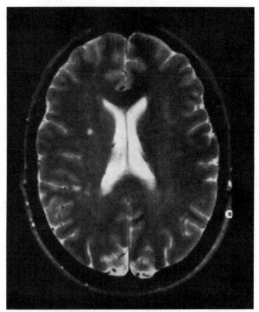

FIGURE 6-18.
A T2-weighted image. Cerebrospinal fluid, having a relatively long T2, appears bright; the substance of the brain, especially the white matter, appears dark because of its shorter T2.

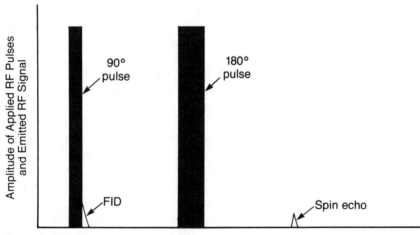

FIGURE 6-19.
Strength of applied and emitted radio frequency (RF) signal. The FID and the 90-degree pulse are sufficiently close in time that recording the FID without contribution from the 90-degree pulse would be difficult. Recording a spin echo without interference from the 180-degree pulse is easier.

the beginning of the recording period were delayed until the pulse signal has entirely died out of the system, a large part of the FID curve would be lost. A spin-echo sequence solves this problem: The spin echo does not even begin until some time after the end of the last applied radio frequency pulse, so that the entirety of the received signal can be used to make an image without being contaminated with large amounts of radio frequency from the pulses. Also, the fact that the apex of the spin echo touches the T2 decay curve, no matter how steep the T2* decay curve (or FID) is, makes it possible to get reasonably strong emitted signals from tissues even in a relatively inhomogeneous magnetic field. Inhomogeneous fields still exact their toll: The area under a spin-echo envelope diminishes as inhomogeneity makes the T2* decay faster, but at least most of the signal-destroying effects of field inhomogeneity can be avoided. For these reasons, some form of spin-echo sequence is used for almost all NMR imaging today.

Let us go back for a minute to our 90-degree–180-degree (or spin-echo) pulse sequence. As we have seen, with extremely short TE values, tissues with different T2 values will look very similar, whereas with very long TE values, little or no spin echo—and hence no useful image—will be possible at all. Therefore, the possibilities are really only two: A very short TE can be used if one desires to make an image without much variation based on T2 differences among tissues or an intermediate value of TE can be used in order to display an image that shows significant T2 differences. In practical terms, these "short" TE times are on the order of 15 to 25 milliseconds, whereas the intermediate values ("long" values in NMR imaging jargon) are on the order of 60 to 130 milliseconds.

But even though these longer TE values are useful to accentuate T2 differences among tissues, it is inevitable that the longer the TE, the lower the amplitude of the spin echoes. And since there is less signal in them from which to make an image, the images made with these long TE values have a lower signal-to-noise ratio than do images with short TE values; they are therefore noisier and can show less anatomic detail. This trade-off is inevitable with T2-weighted MRI; as more T2 differentiation (or T2 weighting) is used, the image noise and unsharpness increase and the anatomic detail decreases. Figure 6-20 shows an image obtained with a short TE and the same structure with a longer TE; notice that all of the parts of the image have become darker as the spin echoes have decreased in magnitude. Figure 6-20C is the same as Fig. 6-20B except that the overall gain of the

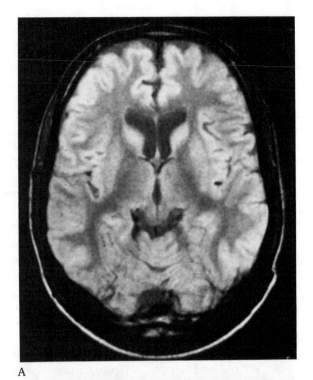

A

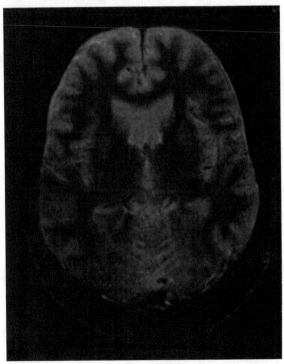

B

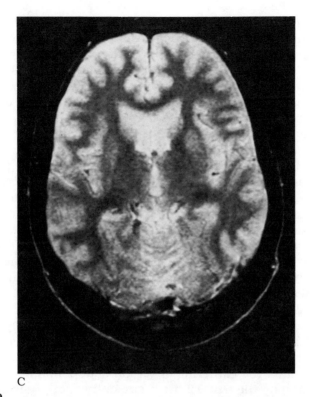

C

FIGURE 6-20.
A. An image obtained with a short TE, and hence little T2 weighting (the image also has little T1 weighting, which we will talk about later, and hence could also be called a "balanced" or "spin-density" image). B. The same patient imaged with a long TE. There is now strong T2 weighting. Notice that the overall signal intensity of the brain has decreased. C. This is the same section as imaged in B, but the overall image brightness has been increased to help visualize the brain.

picture has been increased electronically. Comparing Fig. 6-20A with Fig. 6-20C, it is obvious that Fig. 6-20C contains stronger contrast based on T2 differences among the tissues. It appears that certain structures have gotten brighter. But remember that their signal has not really gotten stronger; the structures merely appear relatively brighter because the overall picture brightness has been increased. Figure 6-20C is the usual way in which T2-weighted images are displayed.

Multiple Spin Echo

Finally, we discuss the multiple spin-echo sequence (see Fig. 6-15). Recall that the time required for complete T2 relaxation to occur is usually considerably longer than the TE employed with most pulse sequences. After the first spin echo (that is, after the spin echo produced by a 90-degree–180-degree pair of pulses), it should be possible to create another spin echo by applying another 180-degree pulse. Remember that the decay of signal after the peak of the spin echo is primarily due to T2* relaxation—that is, it is primarily due to a nonrandom dephasing, which can still be reversed, rather than to the random T2 dephasing, which cannot—and a second 180-degree pulse merely places the transverse magnetization vector of the faster precessing protons behind the slower precessing ones again; they then rephase and another spin echo is produced. Of course, the peak signal in the second spin echo is not as high as the peak signal in the first one, since T2 relaxation has continued to occur, but it is a spin echo all the same, and the signal that comprises it can be used to make an image. In fact, a 90-degree pulse may be followed by many 180-degree pulses, each of which is followed by a spin echo, and each of which may be used to make a separate image. As one might imagine, these images have different degrees of T2 contrast dependence. Also, a multiple spin-echo experiment permits the gathering of several data points from which to estimate the true T2 decay curve; the more such points are acquired, the more accurately the curve can be drawn and the more accurately T2 can be calculated for the imaged tissue.

In summary, the spin-echo pulse sequence can be used to make images in which the gray scale depends on T2 variations in tissues; tissues with long T2 values will tend to look bright and those with short T2 values will tend to look darker. The time from the 90-degree pulse to the receipt of the spin echo is known as TE; images made from pulse sequences with very short TE values have little T2 weighting. Images made with longer TEs reveal more T2 contrast but suffer from increased noise and image unsharpness and decreased spatial resolution. Images cannot be made with extremely long TE values because there is simply not enough available signal from which to construct the image.

Repetition Time

We must now turn to the issue of creating an image in which the gray scale depends on variations from tissue to tissue of their T1 values.

First, we need to review what this relaxation parameter is.

Remember, we defined it as the phenomenon by which a tissue's longitudinal magnetization (that is, magnetization in the Z direction) grows to its ultimate maximum under the influence of a static magnetic field. Remember: Different tissues have different T1 values, the T1 values of most body tissues are measured in hundreds of milliseconds, this growth of tissue magnetization approaches a value asymptotically, and the T1 value is defined as the time required for approximately 63 percent of the magnetization to appear. We have said that, theoretically, T1 relaxation could be observed by instantly applying a static magnetic field to a tissue where none had been applied before, but that this is not feasible. As we will see, this is certainly not the way T1 is measured either in creating NMR images or in other kinds of NMR experiments. In fact, what is done is to perform an entire experiment (or imaging process) while the tissue stays within a constant static magnetic field. What happens is that the tissue's longitudinal magnetization is destroyed, and then grows again, and the rate at which this occurs is measured.

In order to understand how this is done, let us consider a tissue that rests within a static magnetic field and thus has a longitudinal magnetization (see Fig. 6-21). Now let us apply to this tissue a 90-degree radio frequency pulse. The tissue's net magnetization vector is now moved from the Z direction into the XY or transverse plane in which it rotates,

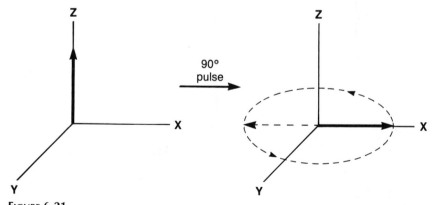

FIGURE 6-21.
Longitudinal magnetization is moved to the transverse plane by a 90-degree pulse. Before any T2 relaxation has taken place, the magnetization in the transverse plane is the same strength as it was prior to being moved out of the longitudinal direction.

70

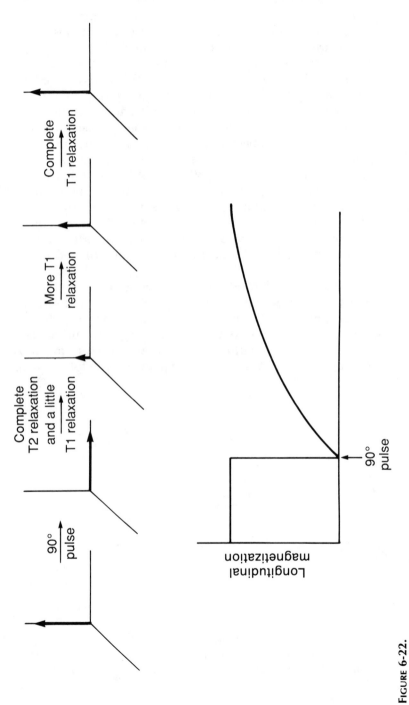

FIGURE 6-22.
Growth of longitudinal magnetization (T1 relaxation) after a 90-degree pulse. Note that immediately after the pulse, there is no longitudinal magnetization, but it immediately begins to grow and ultimately reaches its full value asymptotically.

or precesses, in the manner we described previously. But for the moment let us ignore any transverse magnetization and merely concentrate on the longitudinal (Z) magnetization. Immediately after the radio frequency pulse, there is no longitudinal magnetization at all; that is, the longitudinal magnetization vector has an amplitude of zero. This means that the sum, or net, of the magnetization of all the individual protons within the tissue does not add up to any measurable magnetization in the Z direction. But we must not forget that the main magnetic field is never turned off; therefore, the instant the 90-degree pulse has destroyed the longitudinal magnetization, the magnetic tissues of the individual protons are acted on by the main magnetic field and begin to be pulled back toward the Z direction. As we described previously, this does not happen instantaneously, but exponentially; that is, the regrowth of longitudinal magnetization begins rapidly and then slows, ultimately approaching its original value asymptotically. This process is illustrated in Fig. 6-22.

Meanwhile, of course, any magnetization that had been created in the transverse plane precesses and causes a signal to be emitted. The signal then decays according to the rules of T2 relaxation. But magnetization in the Z direction is not precessing, of course, and does not cause any signal to be emitted; from the point of view of radio frequency signal, its growth is silent.

If Z magnetization and its growth cause no radio frequency signal to be emitted, and if it is the radio frequency signal that is ultimately converted into an image, how do we create an image that reflects T1 relaxation? As with T2-dependent images, T1-dependent images are created by using a series, or sequence, of pulses.

Let us assume that a piece of tissue in a magnetic field is exposed to a series of 90-degree radio frequency pulses. Let us further assume that the time that elapses between the pulses is many times the T1 value of the tissue. Figure 6-23 shows what would be observed. Immediately after each 90-degree pulse, there is no longitudinal magnetization, but this magnetization begins to grow immediately. If one superimposed the growth of the magnetization on Fig. 6-23, Fig. 6-24 would result. But now let us shorten the interval between the 90-degree pulses considerably. If this were done, there would not be sufficient time for a complete recovery of longitudinal magnetization (that is, for T1 relaxation) to occur. The longitudinal magnetization available for each subsequent radio frequency pulse to push into the trans-

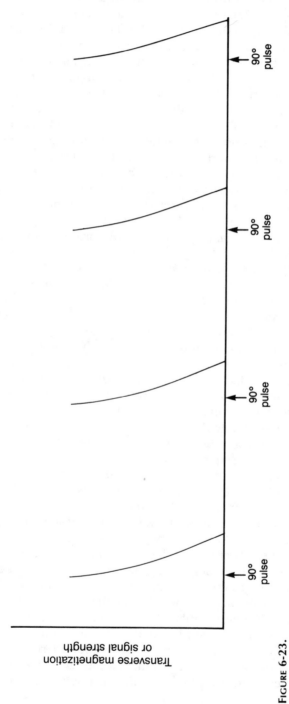

FIGURE 6-23.
What the transverse magnetization would look like if tissue in a magnetic field were exposed to a series of 90-degree pulses. After each 90-degree pulse, transverse magnetization suddenly appears and then decays according to T2*. Since transverse magnetization causes a signal to be emitted, the ordinate in this graph could also be measured in units of emitted radio frequency signal as well as in units of transverse magnetization.

73

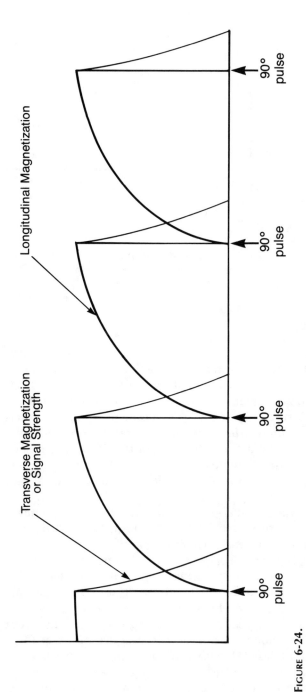

FIGURE 6-24.
Each 90-degree pulse in a series moves the longitudinal magnetization into the transverse plane. T1 relaxation regenerates the longitudinal magnetization between 90-degree pulses; T2* relaxation is the decay of transverse magnetization. The amount of transverse magnetization at the end of each 90-degree pulse is the same (in amplitude) as the amount of longitudinal magnetization at the beginning of the pulse.

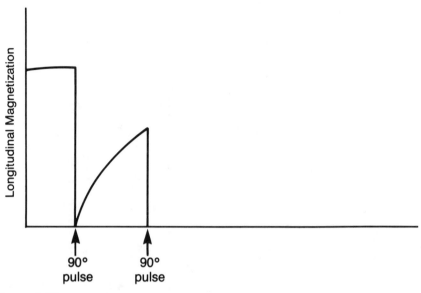

FIGURE 6-25.
Two 90-degree pulses separated by a relatively short period of time. Longitudinal relaxation after the first 90-degree pulse is not complete by the time of the second 90-degree pulse.

verse direction would be smaller than the amount of magnetization that was available for the first pulse (Fig. 6-25).

But now remember that the magnetization in the transverse plane at the end of every 90-degree pulse is exactly the same *in amplitude* as the magnetization in the longitudinal direction was at the beginning of the 90-degree pulse; after all, what the pulse does is merely to change the direction of that magnetization. And if the radio frequency signal that is emitted is proportional to the amplitude of the magnetization in the transverse direction, the radio frequency signal will now be proportional to the amount of longitudinal magnetization that was present at the beginning of each pulse. That is, it will be proportional to the amount of T1 relaxation that has taken place between pulses. Therefore, if a long train of pulses were applied to the tissue, the pulses and the emitted signals might be depicted as in Fig. 6-26.

One can appreciate the consequences of this phenomenon. The shorter the time intervals are between 90-degree pulses, the less T1 relaxation will have taken place (that is, the less the longitudinal magnetization will have had a chance to grow), the less the magnetization will be moved

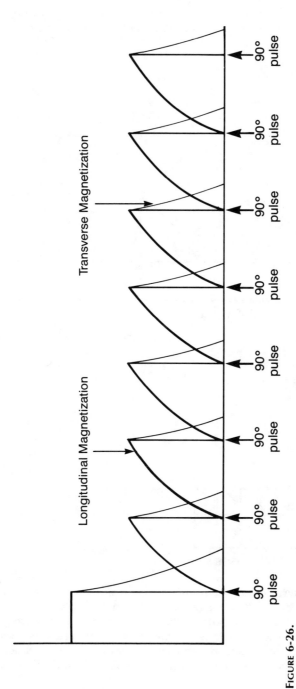

FIGURE 6-26.
A series of 90-degree pulses with short time intervals between them. T1 relaxation is not complete in the interval between the pulses. The amount of transverse magnetization at the end of each 90-degree pulse is the same as the amount of longitudinal magnetization at the beginning of each pulse.

into the transverse plane by each pulse, and the smaller the signal that will be emitted (Fig. 6-27). Conversely, the longer the interval is, the stronger the signal will be after each pulse, at least up to a limit; if the interval between pulses is four or five times the T1 value, the longitudinal magnetization will have recovered between pulses nearly as much as it

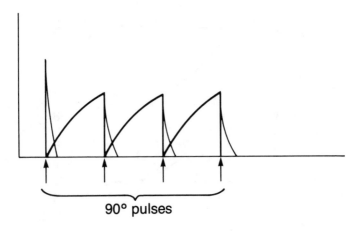

90° pulses

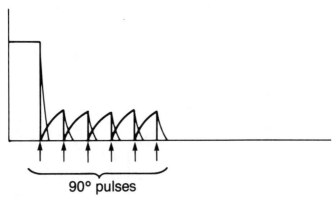

90° pulses

FIGURE 6-27.
At the top, an intermediate amount of time elapses from one 90-degree pulse to the next. The longitudinal magnetization cannot completely recover its original value. At the bottom, the 90-degree pulses appear more frequently. There is even less recovery of longitudinal magnetization (that is, even less T1 relaxation occurs) so that the amount of transverse magnetization that appears immediately after each 90-degree pulse is less than what is shown at the top.

can, and increasing the time interval even further will not permit much more signal to be generated. The time that elapses between 90-degree pulses is known as *TR* (*repetition time*).

Now let us assume that more than one kind of tissue is being imaged. One kind has a long (slow) T1 relaxation and the other, a short (fast) T1. Each of these tissues will be subjected to the same series of radio frequency pulses, but each will *not* have the same amount of longitudinal magnetization growth between each pair of pulses. Therefore, each will have a different amount of magnetization moved into the transverse plane after each pulse and will give off a different strength of signal: The long T1 tissue will have a small amount of magnetization in the Z direction, which, when moved into the transverse plane, will give off a small amount of signal, and the short T1 tissue will have a larger amount of magnetization growth in the longitudinal direction, which will be moved into the transverse direction and thus will give off a stronger signal. Figure 6-28 shows how this might work. And if an image is made using the signals produced by these tissues subjected to these pulses, the long T1 tissue will look relatively dark and the short T1 tissue will look relatively bright (see Fig. 6-29). If TR were very long, virtually complete T1 relaxation would have occurred in all tissues, and there would be no T1-dependent differences in

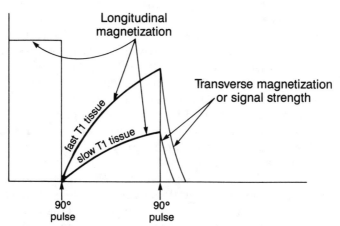

FIGURE 6-28.
Magnetizations of two tissues with different TRs subjected to two 90-degree pulses that are relatively close together. The fast T1 tissue will have relaxed more by the time the second 90-degree pulse appears. Its greater longitudinal magnetization will be converted by the second 90-degree pulse to more transverse magnetization than in the other tissue.

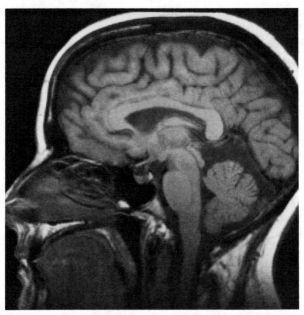

FIGURE 6-29.
T1-weighted image. Most of the contrast depends on the T1 variations among tissues: Tissues with long T1 values appear dark and tissues with short T1 values appear bright.

longitudinal magnetization from tissue to tissue and therefore no differences in T1-dependent transverse magnetization after each radio frequency pulse and no T1-dependent differences in emitted radio frequency signal. Such an image would not have its gray scale affected by T1 variations in the tissue at all. Therefore, relatively short TR values are used to make T1-dependent images in MRI; these values typically range from 200 to 800 milliseconds when imaging at commonly used field strengths. Alternatively, if one wants to make an image with little or no T1 dependence, long TR intervals are used; these are typically on the order of 2,000 milliseconds and may be slightly higher when high-field magnets are used.

Since images made with short TR values exhibit less signal than they would with longer TR values, the signal-to-noise ratio will be worse with short TRs. This is less severe, however, than the signal-to-noise problem caused by long TE values. The ways to compensate for it are discussed later.

In this discussion we have ignored one problem: The radio frequency signal emitted immediately after a 90-degree pulse may be hard to record. Remember that spin-echo pulse sequences were used to solve this problem (as well as to produce T2-dependent images). In fact, what is also usually done in T1-dependent imaging is to generate a spin echo. Here again, the spin echo is produced by applying a 180-degree pulse shortly after each 90-degree pulse, so that the actual pulse sequence used looks something like Fig. 6-30. Figure 6-30A reveals what would happen if the same pulse sequences were used with two tissues with different T1 values. Figure 6-30B is important: It depicts typical pulse sequences in most common current use. Remember that the MRI is made from the recorded signal of the spin echo, and that the brightness of each tissue is proportional to the amplitude of the signal in the spin echo.

Before we proceed to other topics, a few things are worth noting about these spin-echo sequences. One important point is that although certain pulse sequences (those with short TR and TE values) are commonly referred to as T1-weighted sequences and others (those with long TR and long TE values) are usually referred to as T2-weighted images, in fact both types of pulse sequences produce images with some contribution from *both* T1 and T2. Why this is so should be easy to understand. In a T1-dependent image, although TE is relatively short, the TE interval still exists; no matter how short it is, some T2 relaxation can occur during it, and tissues with different T2 relaxation times will have different degrees of relaxation. This effect could be eliminated only if TE were zero, which, in a spin-echo sequence, is impossible. Alternatively, the so-called T2-dependent images, which are those with a long TR and a long TE, could be free of effects from different T1 values in the different tissues *only if* the TR value were so long that *all* tissues had undergone virtually complete T1 relaxation in the TR interval. Since, for those substances with the longest T1 values (such as urine and cerebrospinal fluid), this interval would have to be many seconds long, it is simply not practical to use such a pulse sequence, so that even the T2-weighted pulse sequences usually produce pictures with some T1 weighting.

One may wonder why other pulse sequences are not possible. For instance, why not use a pulse sequence with a long TR and a short TE, or a short TR and a long TE? Consider the former: An image with a long TR and a short TE will have relatively little T1 weighting and relatively little T2 weighting; the only factors remaining that would permit any contrast in the tissues would be mobile proton density (which varies relatively little among soft tissues) and flow;

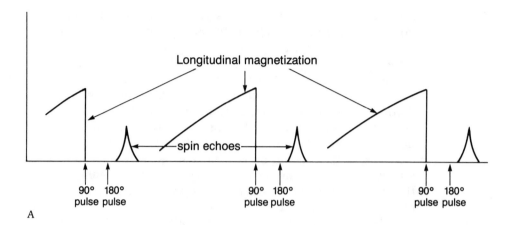

A

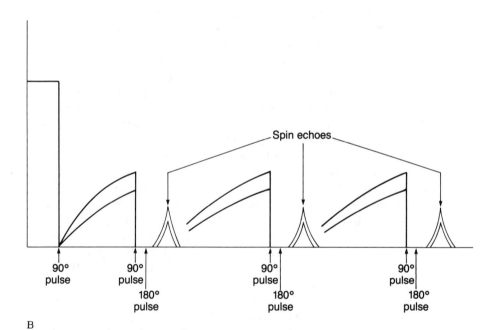

B

FIGURE 6-30.
A. Tissue is exposed to a series of 90-degree–180-degree pulse pairs. Each
180-degree pulse is followed by a spin echo; the amplitude of the spin echo
is determined both by how much longitudinal magnetization was present at
the instant of a 90-degree pulse and by T2 decay. B. Magnetizations of two
tissues with different T1 values are demonstrated: The amplitudes of the
spin echoes are different for the two tissues, and reflect the tissues' different T1 values (the amplitudes of the spin echoes *also* reflect the tissues'
T2 values, but for the purposes of this diagram, the T2 decay rates of the
tissues are assumed to be identical).

such images would have relatively little tissue contrast. Such images are often called proton density images, or spin density images, or "balanced" images (see Fig. 6-20A). Alternatively, the use of a sequence with a short TR and a long TE would produce an image that depended to a considerable degree on *both* T1 and T2. One might first think that this would provide images with very good contrast (after all, this is America, where more is usually better), but things usually do not turn out that way. Among aqueous tissues, tissues that tend to have a long T1 also tend to have a long T2, and since the long T1 tends to make the tissues look darker and the long T2 tends to make the tissues brighter, T1 contrast and T2 contrast tend to work against each other and produce an image whose overall contrast range is not particularly useful. Also, shortening TR and lengthening TE are maneuvers that decrease the amplitude of the spin echo; if they are performed together, the signal-to-noise ratio of the resulting image will be very low.

We now need to discuss proton or spin density a little more. Recall that anatomic parts vary in the amount of hydrogen nuclei they contain: Airways, lung, and intestinal gas contain very little, and thus have negligible magnetization, emit no appreciable signal, and appear dark on all images. Cortical bone, other calcified structures, and certain dense collagenous tissues have more hydrogen nuclei, but have extremely short T2 values and therefore also appear dark. The contrast produced by these dark regions, when they are adjacent to soft tissues and liquids that emit signal, is known as "proton density" weighting or "spin density" weighting. This contrast is, of course, present in images no matter what degree of T1 weighting or T2 weighting is also present. This is an important point: Some of the commonly accepted terminology divides standard images into "T1-weighted," "T2-weighted," and "proton density–weighted," as if these features were mutually exclusive. They are not; there is proton density weighting in virtually all standard images, whether or not T1 weighting or T2 weighting is superimposed. (It is possible to construct images which reflect *only* T1 or T2 differences among tissues, but these are computer-reconstructed images produced by calculating T1 or T2 values for each voxel, using pulse sequences that use at least two TR and two TE values. The relaxation times thus calculated are prone to considerable error for a number of reasons, including the small number of TR and TE values and the inhomogeneity of the radio frequency field. The images thus produced are called *synthetic images*.)

Inversion Recovery

The next pulse sequence we consider is known as the *inversion recovery* sequence. This pulse sequence is especially good at creating images with strong T1 contrast. To understand it, we need to go back to some basics.

Remember that for the spin-echo pulse sequence, the first radio frequency pulse of any group was a 90-degree pulse. This pulse moves longitudinal magnetization into the transverse (XY) plane. It is followed by a 180-degree pulse that moves the magnetization from one place in the transverse plane to another (en route, the magnetization leaves the plane but winds up back in it by the end of the pulse). But now imagine what would happen if the first pulse in a sequence—that is, the pulse applied to tissue whose magnetization is in the longitudinal direction—were a 180-degree pulse. This pulse would move the tissue magnetization out of the longitudinal direction, *through* the transverse plane and ultimately deposit it in the longitudinal axis again but pointing in the opposite direction (Fig. 6-31). The net vector would be in the opposite direction from the initial vector.

Now we need to review a couple of points about this magnetization in the negative longitudinal direction. First of all, it does not cause the tissue to emit any radio frequency signal. Remember that radio frequency signal is *only* emitted when there is some element of magnetization in the transverse plane, which will precess in that plane; after a single

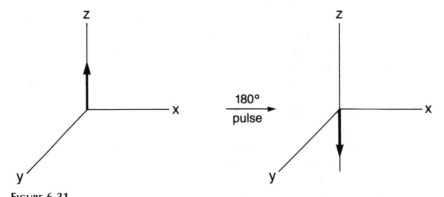

FIGURE 6-31.
The longitudinal magnetization of a tissue will be reversed in direction by a 180-degree pulse. After the 180-degree pulse, the longitudinal magnetization still exists but is pointing in the negative Z direction.

180-degree pulse, there is still no magnetization in the transverse plane. The second important concept is the T1 relaxation that this inverted magnetization undergoes. Remember that after a single 90-degree pulse, there is no magnetization in the Z direction, and that T1 relaxation refers to the growth—or re-growth—of this magnetization (see Fig. 6-22). But if the magnetization has been inverted by a single 180-degree pulse, T1 relaxation also occurs. This might well be expected, since the inverted magnetization is directly opposite to the direction of the main magnetic field. What happens is that the magnetization begins to shrink (Fig. 6-32)

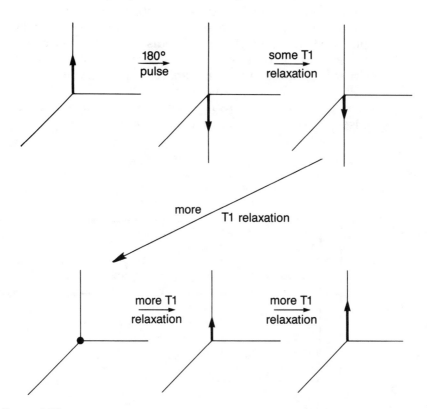

FIGURE 6-32.
The effect of T1 relaxation on longitudinal magnetization after the magnetization has been inverted by a 180-degree pulse. The magnetization increases in the positive Z direction; that is, the magnetization in the negative Z direction first shrinks until it reaches zero, and then positive Z magnetization appears and grows.

and eventually reaches zero magnitude. And of course, it continues to grow after it has reached zero until it ultimately regains its original magnitude. The *rate* at which this magnetization changes (first shrinking and then growing) is exactly the same as the rate at which it would have grown after a single 90-degree pulse. As the magnetization shrinks to zero and then grows, its changing magnitude can be drawn as in Fig. 6-33.

It is important to note that at no time during this process does the net tissue magnetization move into—or appear in—the transverse plane, even though it passes through the plane *during* the 180-degree pulse. It merely shrinks to zero and then grows again, staying in the longitudinal axis the whole time.

But if this magnetization emits no signal, how can we use it to make an image? We do so by subjecting the tissue to a second pulse, this time a 90-degree one, while the T1 relaxation from the first 180-degree pulse is taking place. This second pulse causes any existing longitudinal magnetization to be moved into the transverse plane, where it will begin to precess and cause signal to be emitted. The time interval between the 180-degree pulse and the 90-degree pulse is known as *TI* (for *inversion time*).

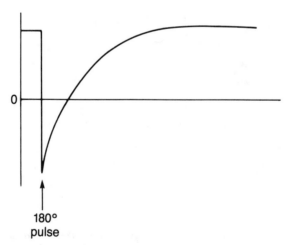

FIGURE 6-33.
This curve reveals the changes in longitudinal magnetization following a 180-degree pulse, and reflects the vectors shown in Fig. 6-32.

One can see what will happen if TI is varied (Fig. 6-34). If the 90-degree pulse follows the 180-degree pulse almost immediately, a strong (albeit negative) longitudinal magnetization will be moved into the transverse plane and a strong signal will be emitted. If the interval is lengthened, the magnetization will have shrunk, so that the magnetization ultimately moved into the transverse plane will be weaker and the resulting signal emitted will be weaker. If the 90-degree pulse is applied at exactly the time at which the magnetization has shrunk to zero, no signal will be emitted. And, as one can easily imagine, the re-growth of magnetization in the (positive) longitudinal direction will permit a signal to be emitted as this magnetization is moved into the transverse plane.

If the strength of the signal after the 90-degree pulse is plotted as a function of TI, the graph will look something like that in Fig. 6-35.

Echo Time and Repetition Time

But now we encounter the same problem that we had when we initially discussed pulses and signals: After a 90-degree pulse, the emitted signal is in the form of an FID, which is hard to record and therefore hard to use to make an image. To get around this, we use the same trick that was used with the standard spin-echo pulse sequence; that is, after the 90-degree pulse, another 180-degree pulse is applied, producing a spin echo (by exactly the same mechanisms that operated in the simple spin-echo sequence) (Fig. 6-36), which in turn is recorded and used to make an image. As with the simple spin-echo sequence, the time between the 90-degree pulse and the receipt of the spin echo is called TE. Since inversion recovery images are usually intended to highlight T1 differences, T2 weighting is usually minimized by using as short a TE as possible.

In summary, then, the usual inversion recovery pulse sequence consists of a 180-degree pulse (the inverting pulse), a 90-degree pulse (which produces an FID that is usually ignored), and a 180-degree pulse, which produces a spin echo that is recorded and used to create an image. This triplet of pulses is repeated many times in the course of creating an image, and in the long string of pulses that results, the

86

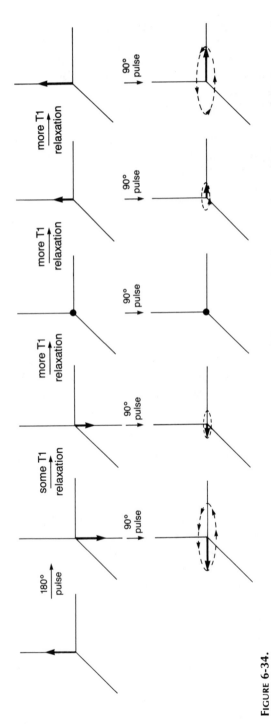

FIGURE 6-34.

The changes of magnetization that occur when tissue is exposed first to a 180-degree pulse and then to a 90-degree pulse. If the time (TI) between the two pulses is quite short, the magnetization will be inverted and then quickly moved into the transverse plane. If the time is a little longer, some T1 relaxation will have taken place, so that the inverted magnetization will have shrunk and a smaller amount of magnetization moved into the transverse plane. If TI is a little longer, and occurs just at the instant in which there is no longitudinal magnetization, the 90-degree pulse will not move any magnetization into the transverse plane at all. As the TI grows still longer and more T1 relaxation has taken place, more and more positive longitudinal magnetization will be moved into the transverse plane by the 90-degree pulse.

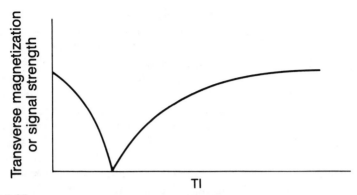

Figure 6-35.
The amount of tissue magnetization that would be moved into the transverse plane (and produce a radio frequency signal) as a function of the interval (TI) between a 180-degree pulse and a subsequent 90-degree pulse. Notice that the *absolute* amount of magnetization in the transverse plane first falls to zero and then rises again as TI lengthens. The value of TI for which the signal strength is zero is known as the "bounce point."

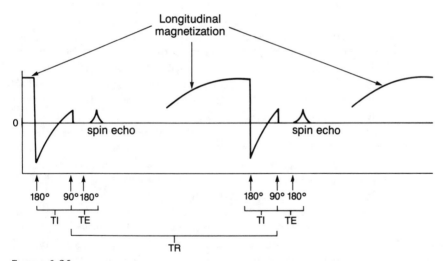

Figure 6-36.
Complete inversion recovery sequence. The longitudinal magnetization and its response to the inverting (180-degree) pulse and the 90-degree pulse is seen. The spin echo that follows the second 180-degree pulse is shown as well.

time interval between successive 90-degree pulses is known as TR, just as it was with the simple spin-echo sequence.

We mentioned that an inversion recovery pulse sequence could be used to make images with especially strong T1 dependence (Fig. 6-37). In order to understand this, we need to go back to a simple spin-echo sequence, and review how TR affects T1 contrast. Let us imagine a situation in which two tissues with different T1 values are being imaged with a standard spin-echo sequence and it is important to distinguish them from one another. We would not want to use a sequence with a very long TR; if we did, both tissues would have undergone complete T1 relaxation between each set of pulses, and would emit the same strength of signal. But if a shorter TR interval were used, the tissues would have relaxed to a degree such that the maximum *absolute* difference in longitudinal magnetization between them would have been reached. The tissues would give off radio frequency signals whose intensity was at a maximum difference, and would therefore appear on the image with a maximum contrast difference. Figure 6-38A shows the TR that would maximize the difference in longitudinal relaxation—and hence in signal strength—between the two tissues.

Now let us look at these same two tissues subjected to an inversion recovery sequence, and let us consider the effect of changing TI. If TI were *very* short, neither tissue would have relaxed much from its completely inverted magnetization, both would have strong magnetizations moved into the transverse plane, and both would give off relatively strong signal and would appear relatively bright on the image. Alternatively, if TI were very long, both tissues would have relaxed completely back into the positive longitudinal direction, and would again have a strong magnetization moved into the transverse plane, and both would appear bright. But if TI were of some intermediate value, such that by the time the 90-degree pulse appeared, one tissue (the one with the slower T1) had relaxed to the point at which its longitudinal magnetization was about zero, and the other relaxed so that its longitudinal magnetization was positive in direction and relatively strong, the two tissues would have a large difference in amount of magnetization moved into the transverse plane, a large difference in the strength of signal given off, and a large contrast difference on the image.

One can see by comparing Figs. 6-38A and B that the *maximum* difference in magnetization (and hence signal strength) between the two tissues is greater using the inversion recovery sequence than with the simple spin-echo sequence. The maximum contrast between two tissues with

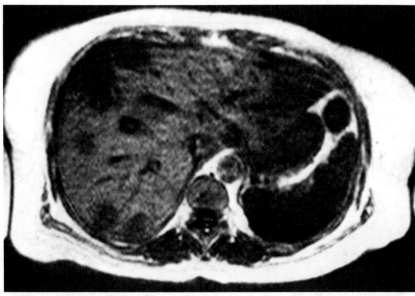

A

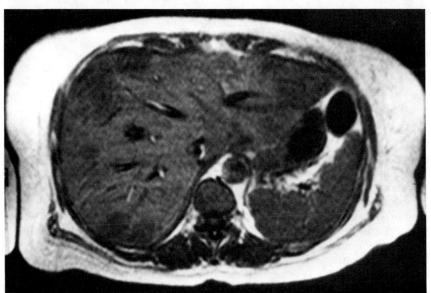

B

FIGURE 6-37.

A. Inversion recovery sequence in a patient with hepatic metastatic carcinoma. The metastases are clearly less intense than the surrounding normal parenchyma, and the spleen is less intense than the normal portions of the liver. Tumor and spleen have longer T1s than does normal liver. B. Standard spin-echo sequence. The contrast between the tumors and the liver, and between the spleen and the liver, is much less striking. The image is less grainy, however; the signal-to-noise ratio is higher.

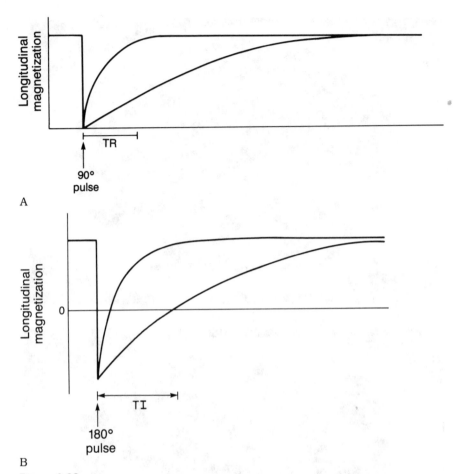

FIGURE 6-38.
A. The longitudinal magnetization changes that two tissues with different
T1 relaxation rates would undergo after a single 90-degree pulse. A particular
TR value that would maximize the absolute difference in longitudinal magnetization between the two tissues is shown. This TR would give the strongest
possible absolute signal difference between the two tissues if a spin-echo
imaging sequence were used. B. The changes in longitudinal magnetization
between the same tissues as those in A if a single 180-degree pulse were
applied. A particular TI value that maximizes the absolute difference in longitudinal magnetization between the two tissues is shown. If an inversion
recovery sequence were used, there would be strong T1 contrast at this TI.

A and B show that the difference in absolute magnetization can be made
greater in B, that is, during inversion recovery imaging. Note in B that if
there were a way to distinguish between positive and negative longitudinal
magnetization, a shorter TI might provide even stronger contrast. Positive
and negative longitudinal magnetization *can* be distinguished by phase differences between the two, so that the potential exists for even stronger T1
contrast.

T1 differences is thus greater with the inversion recovery pulse sequence.

An inversion recovery pulse sequence may produce a peculiar appearance in images, which is sometimes called a *bounce point artifact*. Imagine that the tissue being imaged has a range of T1 values, and imagine that the T1 variation in the tissue blends smoothly from one part of the tissue to another (this might happen in the brain at the gray matter–white matter interface, or in kidney at the corticomedullary junction). Also imagine that the TI is set at such a value that the magnetization of one part of the tissue has not quite relaxed to zero by the time of the 90-degree pulse, whereas the magnetization of the adjacent part of tissue has relaxed through zero and has now reached positive values. Any voxel in the tissue whose average T1 value is such that the longitudinal magnetization is zero at the time of the 90-degree pulse will generate no signal, and the resulting pixel will appear black, whereas the signal strength from nearby voxels whose T1 values are slightly different will be sufficient so that the corresponding pixels will appear gray. Under these circumstances, an image of this tissue may appear to have a black line running through it where no real anatomic surface exists; the black line merely traces the region where the T1 of the corresponding tissue has a specific value (Fig. 6-39).

STIR

In our discussion of the inversion recovery pulse sequence so far, we have shown images formed when TI is long enough so that the longitudinal magnetization is positive by the time the 90-degree pulse is applied; that is, after the inverting pulse, the magnetization of all tissues has relaxed through the shrinking phase, has crossed the point of zero magnitude, and has continued to relax so that it is now oriented in the positive Z direction. Under such circumstances, as we have seen, T1 contrast may be greater than it is with a standard spin-echo sequence, and the polarity of the contrast is unchanged: Short T1 tissues tend to appear brighter than long T1 tissues. But imagine what would happen if TI were so short that the longitudinal magnetization after the inverting pulse never relaxed as far as zero. The 90-degree pulse would transfer longitudinal magnetization in the negative direction into the transverse plane. If this were to happen, the absolute magnetization of tissues with relatively short T1s would be *less* than the absolute longitudinal magnetization of tissues with relatively long T1s; in the re-

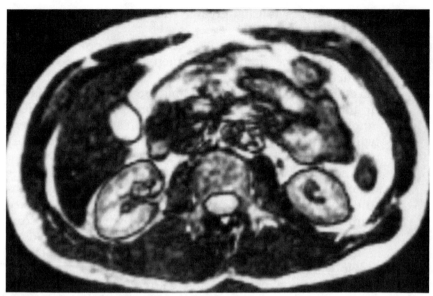

Figure 6-39.
Bounce point artifact. In this inversion recovery image, the voxels at the margins between the kidneys and adjacent fat contain both kidney tissue and fat tissue. Given the particular TI used, the combination of tissues in each of these voxels had a net magnetization of zero, so that the corresponding pixels appear black and form a factitious black line at the outer edge of each kidney.

sulting images, tissues with short T1s would therefore appear darker than tissues with longer T1s. Indeed, if the TI were at the particular value that could catch the magnetization of a given tissue just as it reached zero, that tissue would have no magnetization to be transferred into the transverse plane, would give off no signal at all, and would appear black on the resulting images. This variation of the inversion recovery sequence is often known as a *short TI inversion recovery* (or *STIR*) image.

Such a pulse sequence has been employed for several purposes. First of all, a TI can be chosen so that fat, which usually has the shortest T1 of imaged normal tissues, has a longitudinal magnetization that is at or near zero during the 90-degree pulse (a TI of about 100 milliseconds usually accomplishes this for imaging in intermediate-strength magnets). Since a great deal of the motion artifact that is encountered in some images disappears if the fat gives off no signal, STIR has been used as a motion-suppressing pulse sequence. Also, the reversal of the polarity of T1 contrast in the images is useful: Since focal regions of pathology often have elongated T1s *and* elongated T2s, since tissues with long T2s tend to appear brighter than tissues with short T2s, and since in this pulse sequence tissues with long T1s tend to appear brighter than tissues with short T1s, T1 contrast and T2 contrast reinforce each other (rather than acting against each other, as they do with standard spin-echo sequences). Thus absolute contrast between lesions and their surrounding tissues can be made more distinct. Finally, since lesions can be made to appear very bright against their surrounding background, the sequence may be useful in making visible lesions which, in other pulse sequences, might have been hard to see because of relatively low contrast.

IMAGING PARAMETER CONSIDERATIONS

By this time, we have introduced three terms for independently variable parameters for our pulse sequences: TR, TE, and TI. We need to know what their approximate value should be in order to produce optimal contrast in the images we create.

Let us deal with TE and T2 contrast first. No absolute value is the "best" TE value, but there are some relatively simple rules that guide us in making the proper choice.

First of all, recall that the shorter the TE, the *less* T2 contrast is present. Therefore, in pulse sequences in which T1 contrast only is desired, the TE should be as short as possible. The shortest TE that can be achieved differs from device to device, and from imaging sequence to imaging sequence; in T1-weighted images, TEs ranging from the low teens to about 30 msec have been used. Using the shortest TE possible in T1-weighted sequences not only keeps T2 contrast from cluttering up a T1 image, but also provides the strongest possible signal and hence the best signal-to-noise ratio.

Things get a little more complicated when choosing appropriate TE values for images intended to have good T2 contrast. Recall that the longer the TE is, the greater is the T2 contrast. But this is true only within limits; if the TE is too long, *all* tissues will have had their transverse magnetization decay to negligible levels, so that little contrast—and indeed, little in the way of any interpretable image at all—can be achieved with an extremely long TE. The best possible contrast calls for a TE that depends on the T2 values of the tissues to be distinguished; unfortunately, when setting up an imaging protocol, what the T2 values of the tissues to be distinguished are is usually not known. Indeed, even the general kind of pathology to be encountered may not be predictable, so that choosing the exact TE value that would best show the lesion is usually not possible. And even if one could, the TE values that give the greatest absolute contrast between tissues would probably not be the best ones: Lesion perceptibility is most closely related to the contrast-to-noise ratio of the tissues to be distinguished, so that this factor must be optimized. Ideally, the TE should fall somewhere between the T2 values of the two tissues to be distinguished. Finally, the strength of the magnetic field of the particular machine must be considered: All other things being equal, at any given TE the signal-to-noise ratio tends to be greater with stronger magnets, so that slightly longer TEs can be used at higher fields. Given all these variables, one can see that exact choice of a TE can be difficult, and TEs for T2-weighted images are often chosen empirically. They tend to range anywhere between 60 and 130 milliseconds, with values in the middle of this range most often being useful.

How about TR values and simple spin-echo sequences? As we have seen, long TR values reduce T1 contrast, so that in images intended to be T2-weighted but not T1-weighted, long TR values are usually used. These values are usually chosen so that for most solid tissues, T1 relaxation is nearly complete. Most T1 relaxation has occurred by the time a period corresponding to three times the T1 relaxation time has occurred; given the range of T1 values for most normal tissues, therefore, a TR of about 2,000 milliseconds permits most T1 relaxation to be complete for most tissues. However, materials that have very long T1—such as urine—would require many seconds to elapse if T1 relaxation were to be complete. An extremely long TR would lead to unacceptably long imaging times, however, so that TRs of approximately 2,000 milliseconds are a compromise. This value practically eliminates T1 contrast for most solid tissues, but results in the persistence of some T1 contrast for tissues that have extremely long T1 values.

If a T1-weighted image is desired, choice of TR becomes a little more critical. Remember that the shorter the TR is, the greater is the absolute T1 contrast if T1 contrast is simply defined as the ratio of signal intensities between tissues that are to be distinguished. However, as we have seen, the shorter the TR is, the less is the absolute signal, so that signal-to-noise ratio begins to diminish as TR diminishes. And if we wish to make certain features most easily visible, we must optimize the contrast-to-noise ratio; this is best accomplished by choosing a TR that approximates in value the T1 values of the tissues to be distinguished. The exact value that is best is probably closest to the T1 of the tissue that is to be distinguished and has the longest T1; but, again, we have no way of predicting what this value is in advance. For most solid tissues, therefore, a TR of 400 to 600 milliseconds works well, when using common field strengths. This range is far from exact, however, and both shorter and longer TRs may be effective. And since the T1 values of tissues vary with the magnetic field strength, optimal TRs may be a little longer with high-strength magnets.

In the case of the inversion recovery sequence, choice of a TI interval is also important. When the standard sort of contrast is desired (that is, when short T1 tissues are intended to be brighter), a TI should be long enough that the magnetization of the concerned tissues has crossed the zero point after the inversion pulse, but not so long that the magnetization has reached its completely relaxed state. For most solid tissues, a TI of approximately 400 milliseconds has been found to be useful. For the STIR sequence, a much shorter TI is used, so that the inverted magnetizations of most tissues should have relaxed toward, but not yet reached, the zero point; a TI of approximately 100 milliseconds provides reasonably good contrast; this T1 also enables the magnetization of fat to be approximately zero, which reduces visible motion artifact. TI values much shorter than that permit relatively little T1 relaxation of any tissue, and hence begin to diminish contrast. Longer TIs result in imaging at a time during which some tissues have positive magnetization and others negative magnetization. In this case (if magnitude reconstruction methods are used), contrast becomes very confusing indeed, and the images have not been found to be widely useful. If the inversion recovery has a relatively long TI, so that the polarity of T1 contrast is "standard," as short a TE as possible should be used in order to remove as much T2 contrast as possible. But if the polarity is reversed, as in a STIR sequence, a longer TE can be used, so that T1 contrast and T2 contrast add to each other. A TR value must also be chosen: These values are usually picked to permit complete or nearly complete T1 relaxation after each pulse trio, and values around 2,000 milliseconds or more are often utilized.

CHAPTER 7

Image Generation

So far, we have described the idea that tissue placed in a static magnetic field and subjected to pulses of radio frequency energy can be made to emit a radio frequency signal. That this is true is not brand-new knowledge; the principles were discovered in the late 1940s. What has been more recently developed is the capacity to use these emitted signals to construct an anatomically accurate depiction of the tissues that emitted them. The tricks by which this can be done rest on principles that have been known since the discovery of NMR, but their incorporation into image-making devices has been much more recent.

The receiving antennae that are placed near the patient in an MRI scanning device, and which receive the radio frequency signal emitted from the patient's tissues, provide very little in the way of localizing information from the signal they receive. Anyone who has ever tried to use a radio direction finder on a small boat knows that the ability to pinpoint the direction of a radio frequency signal is fuzzy at best, and to estimate its distance is virtually impossible. The only information that can be directly acquired from the radio frequency signal detected by the antennae is the signal's frequency and amplitude. How, then, can this signal be used to make an accurate image?

Virtually all of the manipulations of the signal that are performed in order to create images depend on the Larmor relationship, which states that the frequency of the signal a tissue absorbs or emits is directly proportional to the strength of the magnetic field in the tissue at the time of the absorption or emission.

97

Before we consider how this works, we should recall the concept of the magnetic field gradient. Remember that the static magnetic field provided by the main magnet is a uniform one in the imaging volume; it is, as much as possible, exactly the same strength from place to place. Also remember that a magnetic field with a gradient can be made; that is, it can be stronger in one place than in another. These gradients are produced within the imaging field by placing coils of wire inside the magnet and running direct current through them. These coils, known as gradient coils, generate small magnetic fields of their own that are added to the main magnetic field to produce gradients. Coils set at angles to each other can, if the current running through them is correctly arranged, make gradients running in any direction. The gradients are linear ones; that is, as one moves from place to place within the magnetic field along the gradient, the change in strength of magnetic field per unit distance will be the same at any location. The entire alteration in magnetic field strength is only a very small fraction of the strength of the main field.

SLICE SELECTION

Radiologists are used to looking at tomographic images, two-dimensional representations of slices of tissue. This is also the ideal way to try to construct an NMR image. But NMR tomographic imaging cannot be performed by subjecting only a slice of tissue to a magnetic field or to a radio frequency pulse; these static magnetic and radio frequency fields simply cannot be shaped so that they are strictly confined to one plane. If we were to place a body part in a magnetic field and subject it to a radio frequency pulse, the emitted signal would come from a large three-dimensional piece of anatomy (Fig. 7-1); this entire signal would be picked up by the radio frequency receiving antenna, and it would be difficult to localize the reconstructed image to one plane. Therefore, a particular trick is utilized by virtually all MRI devices in order to cause only a single tissue slice to emit signal.

Let us suppose that the body part to be imaged is placed in a magnetic field that has a linear gradient (Fig. 7-2); the gradient would be produced by gradient coils as just described. In addition, let us now produce a pulse of radio frequency energy that contains only a single frequency. Remember, the Larmor equation states that radio frequency energy can be absorbed (that is, it can cause the tissue's

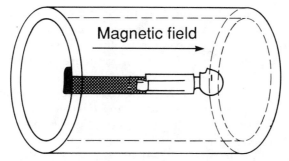

FIGURE 7-1.
Patient placed within a solenoidal magnet. The magnetic field envelopes the entire body. If the body were also subjected to radio frequency pulses of the appropriate frequency, all of the tissues in the entire body would emit signal.

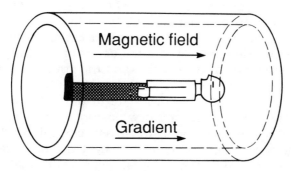

FIGURE 7-2.
The patient lies within a magnetic field with a gradient in a cephalad-caudad axis. If the patient were exposed to radio frequency pulses of just one frequency, signal would be absorbed and emitted only where the field was of a particular strength, which would be in a plane oriented in the transverse direction.

magnetization to precess) only when its frequency corresponds to a particular magnetic field. Therefore, if our pulse contains only a single frequency, even though the pulse passes throughout the volume of the tissue, it will cause the nuclei to change their net angle of precession only where the magnetic field is of a specific value. And if the magnetic field has a gradient, the field will be of that particular value only in one plane. Therefore, our radio frequency pulse of a single frequency will cause the nuclei to change precession angle *only in a particular plane* and subsequently *only the tissue in that plane will emit radio frequency signal*. That emitted signal, once detected by the receiving antenna, contains the information from which the scanner's computer can reconstruct an image, and the image will of course be the image only of tissue in that plane.

In fact, it is impossible to create a very short radio frequency pulse that contains only one frequency; there is inevitably at least a narrow range of frequencies within each pulse. This range of frequencies therefore matches or excites those tissues existing within a narrow range of magnetic field strength; that is, the tissue slice is not really a plane but has a finite thickness. That thickness can be varied by changing either the gradient (the steeper the gradient, the thinner the slice) or the radio frequency pulse (the narrower the band of radio frequency, the thinner the slice).

In order to change the location of the tissue slice, one of two things can be done. If the magnetic field gradient is held constant, merely changing the frequency of the radio frequency pulse slightly will move the plane from its original location to one parallel to it; obviously, the greater the change in frequency is, the greater the distance the plane is moved. Alternatively, the frequency of the radio frequency pulse can be held constant, and the gradient changed; that is, the gradient can be altered so that the plane containing the magnetic field appropriate to the particular radio frequency has moved to a new position. The latter technique is used more commonly in current clinical imaging units.

In addition, the magnetic field gradient can also be changed in direction; that is, instead of going (for example) from a lower to a higher magnetic field as one travels cephalad to caudad in the body, the gradient could be set up so that one travels from a lower to a higher magnetic field as one goes from the right side to the left side of the body, or from the back to the front (Fig. 7-3). It should be obvious, therefore, that the orientation of the plane that is excited by the radio frequency pulse (and ultimately reflected in the image) can be in any direction. Sagittal, coronal, and transverse planes are equally easy to produce, as are planes in angled orientations. Since the method of plane selection is identical no matter what the orientation of the plane, there is no reason why the spatial resolution of an image in one plane need differ from that in an image in another plane. This is quite different from the situation encountered in x-ray CT scanning, where directly obtained images are almost always in the transverse plane, and other planes must be reconstructed from contiguous transverse planes.

MR images may be constructed one plane at a time; that is, enough signal can be made to come from each plane so that the computer has all the information it needs to recon-

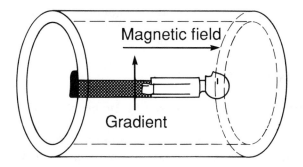

FIGURE 7-3.
The patient now lies in a field with a gradient that exists in the posteroanterior direction. If subjected to radio frequency pulses at an appropriate frequency, the body would absorb and emit radio frequency energy only in a plane oriented in the coronal direction. Radio frequency signals emitted from the patient seen in Fig. 7-2 and here could be used to form tomographic images in the transverse and coronal directions, respectively.

struct an image before another plane is made to emit signal at all. Alternatively, multiple planes may be made to emit signals at once. As we will see, each image requires the application of a large number of pulse pairs (or, in the case of inversion recovery sequences, pulse trios), and a certain amount of time is required between each pair of pulses. During the time period that must elapse between two pulse groups directed toward a particular plane, pulses may also be applied to other planes by quickly changing the gradient (or the frequency of the applied radio frequency pulse); thus the time between pulses is not "wasted" but used to gather data from other planes as well. Later, we will discuss the relationships among imaging time, number of planes in a multislice sequence, and TR.

There also exist techniques so that the emitted signal is not gathered from one plane at once but from an entire three-dimensional volume at once. (Remember, this is just the thing we were trying to avoid by selecting individual slices, but if data from a three-dimensional volume can be collected and subsequently separated into tomographic slices, the same result has been achieved.) Once the emitted signal is acquired, it may be used to reconstruct images in any plane in any orientation within the volume. If the images have the same spatial resolution no matter what their orientation, they are called *isotropic*; if the spatial resolution of images in some orientations is different from that of images in other orientations, the images are said to be *aniso-*

tropic. Isotropic three-dimensional data collection is very time-consuming.

IN-PLANE LOCALIZATION

Although we have now solved the problem of how to get signal to be emitted just from one plane, or slice, we still have to deal with the problem of using the radio frequency signal from that slice to make an anatomically correct tomographic image. Remember, although at this point we know that the signal we record can only have come from one slice, there is still no direct way to tell exactly where the individual portions of the signal arose from within each tissue slice; that is, all of the voxels within the slice emit signals that will be detected all at once, and there is no device (corresponding, for example, to the collimators in a gamma camera) that can be used to determine the source of individual portions of the signal. The solution to this problem again lies in the Larmor relationship.

Remember that in order to select the slice of tissue to be imaged, a magnetic field gradient was turned on during the application of a radio frequency pulse. What now exists through the structure to be imaged is a slice of tissue with nuclear magnetizations precessing in the transverse plane; outside the slice, the remainder of the structure simply retains its longitudinal magnetization, which has not been changed in any way by the pulses. If, during the time that the spin echo is detected and recorded, there is no magnetic field gradient applied, the signal recorded from the spin echo emitted from the plane will be of a single frequency; that is, since the magnetic field is of the same strength everywhere within the plane, the Larmor relationship dictates that the frequency of all the signal emitted from the plane will be the same (Fig. 7-4). But now let us suppose that during the time that the spin echo is produced, another magnetic field gradient is applied. This one will have its vector *perpendicular* to the original slice selection gradient; that is, the new gradient will have its vector lie within the plane whose nuclei are emitting signal (Fig. 7-5). Now, the frequencies of the signal arising from the tissue in various parts of the plane will no longer be the same; rather, the frequency will be higher in the signal emitted from tissue in a stronger magnetic field, and vice versa. All of the emitted signal will be detected by the receiving antenna, and if it were recorded and displayed, it would be apparent that the superimposed multiple fre-

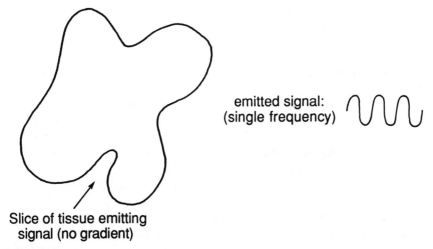

emitted signal:
(single frequency)

Slice of tissue emitting
signal (no gradient)

FIGURE 7-4.
A tomographic slice of tissue in a magnetic field emitting a signal after a 90-degree and a 180-degree pulse. The signal is a single frequency, and is proportional to the strength of the magnetic field.

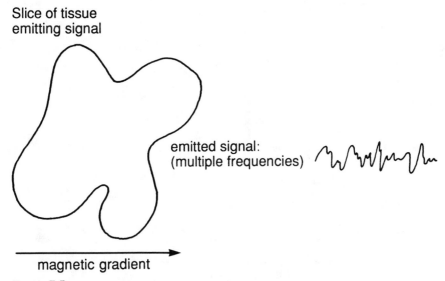

Slice of tissue
emitting signal

emitted signal:
(multiple frequencies)

magnetic gradient

FIGURE 7-5.
A tomographic slice of tissue emitting radio frequency signal in a magnetic field after a 90-degree and 180-degree pulse. In the presence of a magnetic gradient, the field strength varies throughout the slice, and the emitted signal contains a wide range of superimposed frequencies.

quencies would produce a radio frequency waveform that
looks very complex.

Frequency Encoding

A brief diversion is now necessary. Remember from our earlier discussion that a waveform containing multiple frequencies can be subjected to a process called Fourier analysis,
which permits the display of the waveform in such a way
that the *amplitude* of each portion of the signal at a given
frequency can be plotted against the frequency itself, such
as in Fig. 3-8.

Let us see how this might apply to the signal arising from
our plane of tissue. Assume that the plane of tissue is not
homogeneous, but contains three areas that emit particularly strong signal. These areas exist in different positions
along the magnetic field gradient (Fig. 7-6), and thus emit
signal of different frequencies. The signal from all of these
areas mixed together might look dauntingly complex, but,
once subjected to Fourier analysis, the signal from each region would separate out into a specific frequency distribution, and look something like Fig. 3-8.

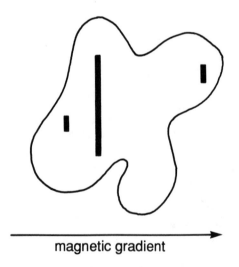

magnetic gradient

FIGURE 7-6.
Tomographic slice of tissue. If we only consider the signal emitted by the
three rectangular portions of tissue within the slice, the signal emitted will
be of three different frequencies. The specific frequencies will be a function
of the position of the portions of tissues along the gradient, and the strength
of each portion will be a function of the amount of tissue in each region. The
combined emitted signal could look like that seen in Fig. 3-8.

Now it may be becoming clear how some of the spatial information needed to construct a tomographic image is acquired. The location of tissue along the gradient determines its frequency; hence, the imager's computer will have the capacity to "assign" the signal from any region of the imaged slice to regions of the tomographic image by correlating the location in the image with a particular frequency.

The gradient that is applied to permit this process is known as the *frequency-encoding gradient*, or the *read-out gradient*, and it is, at least in simple imaging schemes, the last gradient to be applied for any group of pulses. There are two limitations to the use of this gradient: one results in an imaging artifact and the other requires the addition of an entirely new process to create an image.

First the artifact. We have noted that the computer assigns the signal to a particular location in the image by virtue of the frequency of that signal, and can do so since the frequency is a direct function of the local magnetic field, as required by the Larmor relationship. But it turns out that other factors, in addition to the applied static magnetic field and the magnitude of the gradient, control the magnetic field in which each nucleus finds itself. The magnetic field around a proton, or hydrogen nucleus, is determined in a very local sense by the magnetic field generated by charged particles—particularly orbiting electrons—that are close to it, and the particles that most effectively change the magnetic field around a proton are the particles within the proton's own molecule. Since protons within water molecules find themselves in a slightly different magnetic field from protons within lipid molecules, they precess and emit signal with a slightly different frequency than the signal emitted from protons in lipid. (Indeed, the alterations in frequency of emitted signal caused by the location of nuclei within molecules form a large part of the primary basis of the science of NMR spectroscopy, which is an extensive field and totally beyond the scope of this text.) But the computer that sorts out the signals has no intrinsic way of knowing whether the signals come from protons in water or protons in fat. The computer program simply assumes that variations in frequency are produced by variations in spatial location. Therefore, the signal produced by a proton in a fat molecule will, because of its different frequency, be interpreted by the computer as arising from a position in a slightly different magnetic field, that is, slightly farther along the magnetic field gradient. When the computer assigns the signal from fat to a particular place in the image, the signal will always be misregistered on the image in the direction of the magnetic field gradient. This misregistration causes a particular artifact. Since the fat signal is placed on the image in a position slightly shifted from the water signal, where signal from fat moves into an area in which water signal has already been located, the resulting local image is particularly bright. Where the fat signal moves away from an interface with signal from watery tissue, a void is produced in which no signal is assigned by the computer, and a dark region appears. Therefore, wherever there are interfaces between watery tissues and fat tissues on these MR images, this artifact appears; if the water is on one side of the fat, the interface will appear as a factitious bright line, whereas if the water is on the other side of the fat tissue, the interface will appear as a factitious dark line (Fig. 7-7).

These *chemical shift artifacts* can usually be easily recognized, since they are always produced by a slight shift in location of signal in the direction of the frequency-encoding gradient. Their width, and hence their visibility, is greater in images from higher field magnets. They can be made thinner by making the frequency-encoding gradient steeper, but only at the cost of diminishing the signal-to-noise ratio.

But the main problem with the frequency-encoding gradient is that it permits the computer to sort out the signals coming from the imaged tissue slice only in one axis; bits of

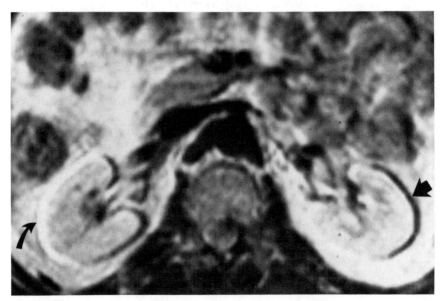

FIGURE 7-7.
Chemical shift artifact. Note the black line (arrow at right) where the lateral edge of the left kidney abuts the adjacent fat, and the white line (arrow at left) where the lateral edge of the right kidney abuts the adjacent fat.

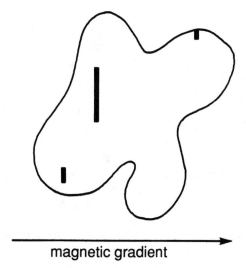

magnetic gradient

<small>FIGURE 7-8.</small>
The three regions of tissue vary in location, but are at the same places along the magnetic gradient. The signal they emit will be indistinguishable from that in Fig. 7-6 and Fig. 3-8.

tissue in the imaged plane that are positioned along an axis perpendicular to the frequency-encoding gradient all have the same frequency and would, unless something else were done, be indistinguishable in position (Fig. 7-8). One's first idea might be simply to add a simultaneous magnetic field gradient in this new direction, but further thought will show that two gradients simultaneously applied in different directions within the plane will simply add up to a third gradient, the sum of the first two, which leaves us with the same problem. Put another way, there is no single gradient, or simultaneous combination of gradients, that will allow each voxel within the imaged slice to exist within a unique magnetic field and hence to emit signal at a unique frequency. (An imaging technique known as echo-planar imaging can deal with this problem, but is not in current widespread use.)

Phase Encoding

Encoding of spatial information in the imaging plane in the direction at right angles to the frequency-encoding direction is usually accomplished by a process known as *phase encoding*. Imagine that another gradient is transiently applied, after the slice-selection gradient has been turned off but before the frequency-encoding gradient has been turned on. The vector of this gradient, like the frequency-encoding gradient, lies in the imaging plane but is oriented at right angles to the frequency-encoding gradient. This gradient is applied while the protons' magnetizations are precessing in the transverse plane and, like the frequency-encoding gradient, causes the protons to precess at different speeds in different parts of the plane. But this gradient is applied only briefly. When it is turned off, the protons' magnetizations all begin to precess again at the same frequency, but, since they have precessed at different frequencies for a short period, they now precess with slightly different phases (Fig. 7-9). Following this maneuver, the frequency-encoding gradient is turned on, and the spin echo is recorded and subjected to Fourier transformation. Now we are well on the way to being able to assign the signal from each voxel to its appropriate pixel: The voxels emit signals that differ in frequency along one direction in the image, and that differ in phase along another direction in the image. Each voxel thus emits signal that has a unique combination of phase and frequency, and thus the information to assign the signal from each voxel to its appropriate pixel has begun to be available.

It turns out, for standard imaging techniques, that recording a single spin-echo signal from the entire plane does not provide enough information completely to reconstruct the image. Instead, it is necessary to produce as many spin echoes as there are voxels (or pixels) in the phase-encoding direction. For each spin echo, the transient phase-encoding gradient must have a different magnitude. This rule does *not* apply to the frequency-encoding direction in the imaged plane (a single spin echo, acquired during a frequency-encoding gradient and subjected to Fourier transformation, would provide enough information to sort out the signal along the frequency-encoding direction), but it is hard to avoid in the phase-encoding direction. An image whose pixel array is 512×512 will therefore require the creation and recording of 512 spin echoes; if the image were 128×256 pixels, the image would require 128 spin echoes if the phase-encoding direction were in the direction of 128 pixels, or 256 spin echoes if the phase-encoding direction were in the direction of the 256 pixels. Computer tricks can reduce somewhat the number of spin echoes that are required, but these tricks are applied at the cost of a slight loss in spatial resolution.

Chemical shift artifacts that may occur in the frequency-encoding direction do not appear in the phase-encoding direction, but visible motion artifacts are almost always more pronounced in the phase-encoding direction. Most modern

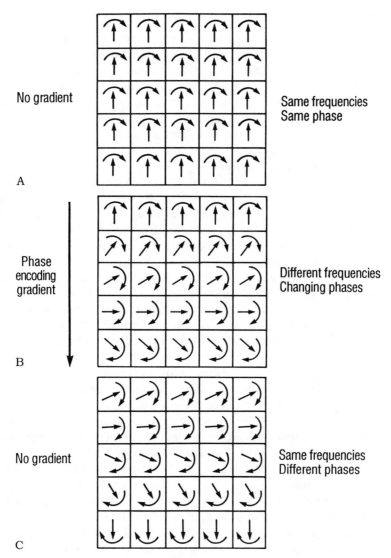

No gradient

Same frequencies
Same phase

A

Phase
encoding
gradient

Different frequencies
Changing phases

B

No gradient

Same frequencies
Different phases

C

FIGURE 7-9.

A. Tomographic slice of tissue, with a 5 × 5 voxel array. Each straight arrow represents the phase of the precessing spins in the voxel, and each curved arrow represents the direction and speed of precession. If there is no gradient, the magnetizations of each voxel precess with the same frequency and stay in the same phase. B. If a phase-encoding gradient is applied, the magnetizations in the lower rows precess at a greater frequency than those in the upper rows, so that with time the phases of the horizontal rows differ more and more. C. If the phase-encoding gradient is turned off, the magnetizations in the voxels now precess at the same frequency again, but the magnetizations in the rows stay at different phases from each other. The phase of each precessing magnetization now uniquely localizes the magnetization in the phase-encoding direction. The signals from the voxels in the direction at right angles to the phase-encoding direction are all the same, however, and could only be distinguished if a subsequent frequency-encoding gradient were applied, perpendicular to the phase-encoding direction, in which case each voxel would have a unique combination of frequency and phase.

imaging devices permit the frequency- and phase-encoding directions to be switched to get the best image.

Another artifact may appear as a consequence of using the phase-encoding gradient. Imagine that one wished to scan only a small part of the body in a particular plane; for example, in a transverse view, one might wish to scan only the spinal canal. The phase-encoding and frequency-encoding gradients would both have to be quite steep (or strong) in order that the canal fill the entire image. The gradients, of course, continue beyond the imaged portion of the transverse slice into adjacent tissue. In the frequency-encoding direction, this does not cause a problem: Signal coming from tissues outside the spinal canal in the frequency-encoding direction can be eliminated simply by discarding all signal with frequencies higher or lower than the range that encompasses the spinal canal itself. But suppose that the gradient in the phase-encoding direction is sufficiently steep that the linear dimension of the spinal canal in the phase-encoding direction involves a net phase shift of 360 degrees. Outside this region, the phase shift will be of greater magnitude, but it is difficult for the computer to distinguish a phase shift of 10 degrees from a phase shift of 370 degrees. Therefore, when the computer reconstructs the image, it will place a bit of anatomy 370 degrees away from the center in the same place as a bit of anatomy 10 degrees away from the center, so that images of anatomic parts outside the desired image area will be superimposed on the anatomy within the region. This is known as *wraparound artifact*, and may be encountered whenever one tries to "cone down" the image to an area that is much smaller than that filled by all body parts in the same plane. Some imaging devices have mechanisms that can eliminate phase wraparound artifact.

To summarize, a standard image in one plane is usually acquired by transiently applying a slice-selection gradient (whose vector is perpendicular to the imaged plane) during the application of the radio frequency pulses. The slice-selection gradient is then turned off and followed by a transient phase-encoding gradient, which is also turned off and followed by a frequency-encoding gradient, which is applied during the recording of the spin echo. The number of pixels in the phase-encoding direction is usually the same as the number of spin echoes that are recorded, and each phase-encoding gradient has a different magnitude, so that there are as many different strengths of phase-encoding gradient as there are pixels in the phase-encoding direction.

Since this technique determines the number of spin echoes that must be recorded, and since the time that elapses

between spin echoes is TR, TR becomes an important deter-
minant of required imaging time. We will discuss the group
of things that together control imaging time subsequently.

MOTION ARTIFACTS AND COMPENSATIONS

So far, our discussion of image reconstruction has depended
on the notion that the imaged tissue remains stationary as
the pulses are being applied and the spin echoes are being
collected. Often, of course, the tissue may move: The patient
may shift position, cardiac muscle contracts and moves,
large vessels pulsate, cardiac contraction is reflected in cerebrospinal fluid pulsation, and respiratory and peristaltic
motion occur. The effects that tissue motion have on the
image are far from simple, and a complete discussion of
them is beyond the scope of this text. Nevertheless, there are
some features of tissue motion effects that should receive
some attention.

First of all, regular repeated motions, such as those produced by the beating heart, by pulsating great vessels, and
by the respiring chest, may produce a kind of "ghosting"
artifact. Imagine, for example, a patient rhythmically breath-
ing every 3 seconds during a scan. If the TR were $1\frac{1}{2}$ seconds, at the start of each data acquisition, the patient's anterior chest wall would be at either of two different points in
the respiratory cycle. The signal from the anterior chest wall
would thus be registered at one of two positions in the
phase-encoding direction, and the image of the chest wall
would appear in two locations, one of which would appear
as a "ghost." Of course, cardiac and respiratory motion
would never be so regular that positions occupied by the
moving structures would only be in a small number of fixed
positions within the imaging cycle; therefore, actual clinical
images show multiple "ghost" artifacts from these moving
structures. In the frequency-encoding direction, both regular and irregular motions tend not to show discrete ghost
artifacts, but simply tend to produce a blurring, or image
unsharpness, which is usually less noticeable than the
ghosts seen in the phase-encoding direction.

There are several ways to compensate for these motion
artifacts. The most obvious but most difficult technique
would be to acquire all of the signal necessary to make an
image in such a short period of time that negligible motion
occurred. Advanced techniques provide image data acquisition in a fraction of a second, but these are not in current
widespread clinical use. Other methods (these include the

use of short TR, small flip-angle gradient–echo imaging, which is discussed later) permit data acquisition sufficiently fast that enough information can be acquired for an image during a single breathhold, which at least eliminates the effects of respiratory motion. Alternatively, multiple sets of imaged data can be acquired and added together to create a single image. When this technique is used, although the "ghosts" still appear, there are so many of them in so many different locations that they begin to combine to form a more uniform and less bothersome blur, rather than remaining as eye-catching discrete imaging features. Alternatively, the tissue motion itself may be suppressed: The patients can be counseled to reduce voluntary motion as much as possible, drugs that temporarily inhibit peristalsis can be administered, fetal motion can be suppressed by maternal administration of sedatives, or one can limit one's practice to Egyptian archeology and image only motionless mummies.

Another approach to suppressing artifact from rhythmic motion is gating of imaging acquisition. Either respiratory motion (monitored by a bellows fastened around the chest) or the cardiac cycle (monitored by sensors of blood flow, blood pressure, or an electrocardiographic signal) can be used to trigger the acquisition of image data. Whatever the triggering device, it is used to initiate a 90-degree–180-degree pulse, spin-echo sequence at a given time (or series of times) within the cardiac or respiratory cycle. Although misregistration of the moving tissue is thus avoided, gated triggering of the pulses and echoes inevitably means that TR is controlled by the heart rate or respiratory rate. To a great extent, then, image contrast is determined by pulse or respiratory rate rather than by free choice of TR by the operator of the imaging device.

MULTISLICE IMAGING

We have discussed the concept of TR, and introduced the idea that a specific number of spin echoes is necessary in order to form an image, so that the product of TR and necessary number of spin echoes establishes a lower limit of time necessary to gather data to create an MR image. But, for the usual spin-echo sequence, in a situation in which only a single slice is being imaged, most of this time is "empty"; that is, TE is quite short compared to TR, and the lengthy period of time that elapses between a spin echo and the next 90-degree pulse is occupied only by T1 relaxation: No further pulses fill this time (Fig. 7-10). In order to make imaging

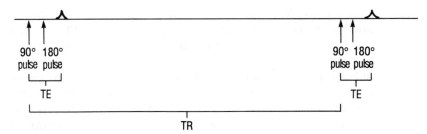

FIGURE 7-10.

A spin-echo sequence applied to a single slice of tissue. With a TR much longer than the TE, a long time elapses between a spin echo and the next 90-degree pulse.

more time-efficient, a common maneuver is used to employ this time to perform a multislice sequence.

Let us assume that five parallel tomographic slices are desired, and that a TR and TE have been selected. Let us assume also that the first slice-selection gradient selects the first slice in the series. A 90-degree pulse is applied, followed by a 180-degree pulse, which is followed in turn by a spin echo. Immediately after this spin echo, the slice-selection gradient may be turned on with a slightly different value, that is, in such a way that the next slice is selected. This second slice can then be subjected to a 90-degree–180-degree spin-echo sequence, after which the third slice is selected, and so forth (Fig. 7-11). In the time that has elapsed

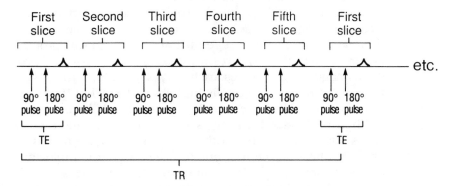

FIGURE 7-11.

Multislice spin-echo sequence. Each pair of pulses follows the preceding spin echo by a very short time, and *is applied to a different* slice. (The slices are determined by different values of the slice-selection gradient.) It should be apparent that the longer the TR is, the more slices can be imaged. The order of application of pairs of pulses to the slices can be varied.

between the first spin echo from the first slice and the second 90-degree pulse *experienced by the first slice*, a spin echo has been elicited from all of the other slices, with no loss in total time. The process is then repeated many times, of course, since each slice must have multiple spin echoes elicited from it, but the total time required to image all of the slices is still no greater than that which would have been required to image just one slice. This trick is in routine use today, and provides the so-called *multislice imaging capacity* of most modern imaging devices.

It should be obvious that the TR controls the amount of time between the end of any spin echo and the next 90-degree pulse for any slice, and thus controls the amount of time available to elicit spin echoes from other slices before the original slice needs to be pulsed again. Since a finite amount of time is needed for the gradients to be switched on and off and the pulses to be generated and the echoes to be recorded, there turns out to be a fixed relationship between the TR and the number of slices that can be included in a multislice imaging technique: *The longer the TR is, the more slices can be imaged simultaneously.*

Multislice imaging with MRI, as with CT, can lend itself to three-dimensional imaging simply by performing contiguous slices. But MRI may also be used to acquire three-dimensional images directly. The slice selection process is eliminated, and the entire three-dimensional volume of tissue to be imaged is subjected to radio frequency pulses. Spatial localization of the resulting array of voxels is accomplished by using two successive orthogonal phase-encoding gradients and a subsequent frequency-encoding gradient perpendicular to both of them; the resulting emitted radio frequency signal is subjected to a process called *three-dimensional Fourier transformation*. Although this process is time-consuming, the resulting data can be used to produce images whose planes are in any orientation, whose spatial resolution can be equally high no matter what the plane orientation, and whose signal-to-noise ratio is high.

When multislice imaging is performed, the gaps among slices may be varied in width. If very narrow gaps are used, or if the slices are contiguous, a problem that is important to know about arises. Remember that the thickness of each slice is determined by the steepness of the slice-selection gradient and the frequency range of the radio frequency pulses. But, as we already learned, it is not possible to generate a short pulse whose range of frequencies is very precisely defined; instead, each pulse contains a small amount of energy whose frequencies are above and below the intended frequency range. This means that the pulses will have effects on tissue adjacent to the slice that is intended to be imaged by each pulse pair (or, in the case of an inversion recovery sequence, by each pulse trio). And if this tissue falls into the volume included by an adjacent slice, the result is that the tissue magnetization of each slice is affected not only by the pulses intended for it, but also by the pulses from adjacent slices. This, in turn, is the equivalent of shortening the TR for each slice, which in turn increases the amount of T1 weighting. The unintentional increase in T1 weighting may not cause much of a problem if T1 weighting is desired in the first place, but in T2-weighted images in which T1 weighting is to be avoided, this artifact may significantly degrade the final images. In addition, the "spillover" effect of pulses from adjacent slices inevitably diminishes longitudinal magnetization, so that the signal from each slice is diminished. These deleterious effects may be lessened by interleaving the slices—that is, by designing the imaging device so that pulses are not intended to affect adjacent slices sequentially—but they cannot be entirely eliminated. Therefore, in T2-weighted images in which it is important to maximize signal-to-noise ratio and minimize T1 weighting, contiguous slices or very small slice gaps should be avoided.

CHAPTER 8

Small Flip Angles and Gradient Echoes

So far in this text, we have limited our discussion of imaging to that of the spin-echo type. This involved first subjecting the sample to a 90-degree radio frequency pulse and then a 180-degree radio frequency pulse to generate a spin-echo signal, which can then be processed for image generation. Recently it has become apparent that it is possible to image in many other ways. In this section we discuss one of these new techniques.

USING SMALL FLIP ANGLES

Just as it is possible to excite a sample with a 90-degree radio frequency pulse to produce transverse magnetization (Fig. 8-1A), it is equally possible to excite the sample with a radio frequency pulse that is less than 90 degrees. For example, the sample could be excited with a 20-degree radio frequency pulse. This means that the sample would lose very little of its longitudinal magnetization, rather than losing all of it as it would with a 90-degree radio frequency pulse. Imagine that if the sample is excited with a 20-degree pulse and only loses a small part of its longitudinal magnetization, and then undergoes longitudinal relaxation, it will take less time to achieve most of its initial longitudinal magnetization again. Recall that with routine spin-echo imaging, we had to wait a significant amount of time to allow the sample to regain longitudinal magnetization so that with a subsequent 90-degree pulse, there would be sufficient transverse magnetization to yield enough signal. Typically, this would

117

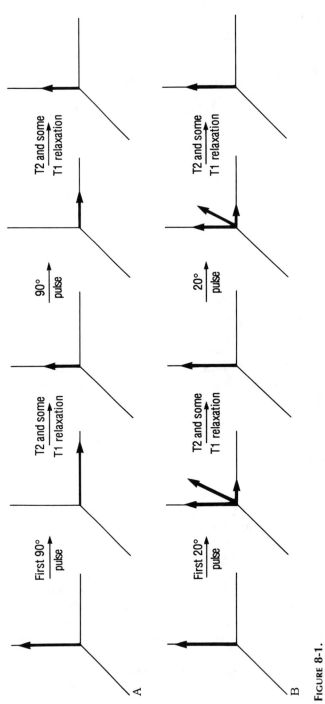

FIGURE 8-1.

A. The magnetization of tissue subjected to two 90-degree pulses. Each 90-degree pulse moves all of the available longitudinal magnetization into the transverse plane. TR is sufficiently short that not all of the original longitudinal magnetization is recovered before the second 90-degree pulse. B. Magnetization of the same tissue subjected to two 20-degree pulses. Immediately after each pulse, most of the longitudinal magnetization is still present. Notice that the transverse magnetization after each pulse is considerably smaller than it was after the application of a 90-degree pulse, and that the amount of longitudinal magnetization present at the time of the second (and any subsequent) 20-degree pulse is greater than it was when 90-degree pulses were used.

necessitate using TR intervals in the range of 300 to 800 milliseconds for T1-weighted imaging and TR intervals in the range of several seconds for T2-weighted images. But if the sample is excited with a pulse much smaller than 90 degrees, in a very short time it will have considerable longitudinal magnetization, so that it becomes possible to do routine clinical imaging with very short TR intervals. Figure 8-1B demonstrates the effect of using partial flip angles on longitudinal magnetization. The smaller the flip angle, the more quickly the sample can regain its longitudinal magnetization.

Let us consider two samples of tissue with different longitudinal relaxation times that are subjected to radio frequency pulses. Figure 8-2A shows what might happen to them if they are subjected to successive 90-degree pulses with a relatively short TR. At the time of each pulse, the tissues have quite different amounts of longitudinal magnetization. But if smaller pulses are used—for example, 20-degree pulses—the longitudinal magnetization of the tissues will behave quite differently, as is seen in Fig. 8-2B. Note that immediately after each pulse, the longitudinal magnetization is still quite strong. Of the longitudinal magnetization that has been destroyed by each pulse, the same *fraction* is regained in the intrapulse interval as was regained after the 90-degree pulses. But the fraction of longitudinal magnetization that is destroyed by each pulse is different in the two circumstances: With a 90-degree pulse, 100 percent of the longitudinal magnetization is destroyed, whereas with the 20-degree pulse, very little is destroyed. Therefore, with repeated 20-degree pulses, eventually a steady state is reached in which both tissues have an average longitudinal magnetization that is pretty close to the maximum.

This situation has a couple of consequences. First of all, even though the TR is very short, the amount of longitudinal magnetization at the beginning of each pulse (which can, at least in part, be moved by the pulse into the transverse plane) is considerably larger than it would be if 90-degree pulses had been used. Also, the *relative* difference in longitudinal magnetization between the two tissues is quite small, so that if images are formed, there will be relatively little T1 contrast. Therefore, if a TE is selected to provide adequate T2 contrast, the resulting image will have relatively strong T2 weighting and very little T1 weighting. Here is one of the major advantages of a short-TR, small-flip-angle pulse sequence: T2-weighted images can be acquired with a relatively short TR, and hence a much shorter imaging time

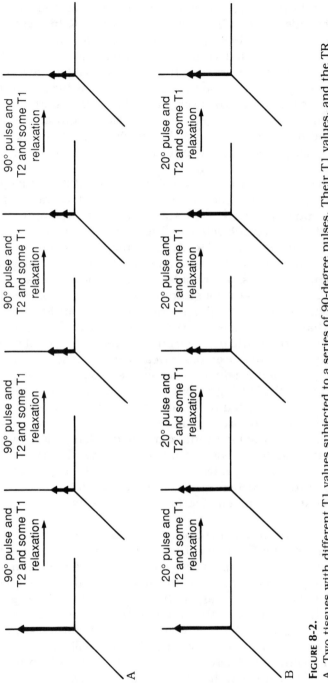

FIGURE 8-2.

A. Two tissues with different T1 values subjected to a series of 90-degree pulses. Their T1 values, and the TR used, result in longitudinal magnetization prior to the second (and any subsequent) 90-degree pulse being relatively small; the magnetizations of the two tissues are different from each other. B. The same two tissues subjected to a series of 20-degree pulses using the same TR. Note that the amounts of longitudinal magnetization prior to the second (and any subsequent) 20-degree pulse is considerably larger than it was when 90-degree pulses were used, and that the differences in magnetizations between the two tissues is relatively small.

than is possible with long TR sequences using 90-degree pulses. Using flip angles at or near 90 degrees reintroduces T1 weighting if the TR is kept short.

Of course, Mother Nature cannot be cheated in MRI any more than she can in any other endeavor, so there are deleterious consequences for using a small flip angle in order to do fast imaging. First of all, if a small flip angle is used, only a small amount of the longitudinal magnetization is ever transferred to the transverse plane. Using any given pulse, the amount of transverse magnetization produced by that pulse relates to the sine of the pulse angle. With a 90-degree pulse, the transverse magnetization produced is 100 percent of the longitudinal magnetization, whereas for a 20-degree pulse, the transverse magnetization produced is much less. With small flip angles, the transverse magnetization is relatively small, so that the signal ultimately emitted by the tissue is relatively low, and the signal-to-noise ratio is relatively low as well. A practical trade-off thus appears: In order for small-flip-angle, short-TR imaging to be useful (and it is primarily useful in permitting quite fast imaging and thus reducing motion artifact), it must suffer from a relatively low signal-to-noise ratio.

GRADIENT ECHOES

In standard spin-echo imaging, the 90-degree pulse is followed by an 180-degree pulse, the latter of which is intended to cause a spin echo. With small-flip-angle imaging, it is common to use another mechanism to produce the spin echo. This is alternatively known as a *gradient echo*, a *gradient-recalled echo*, a *fast field echo*, and other names (these are various manufacturers' terms for the same process). In brief, this amounts to a substitution of a reversed magnetic field gradient for the 180-degree pulse. That is, after the 90-degree pulse (or a smaller pulse), instead of using a 180-degree pulse, the direction of the last magnetic field gradient in the imaging sequence is reversed. This maneuver produces a kind of spin echo. Why this echo should appear may not be immediately obvious; in order to understand it, we need to go back to some fundamental issues.

Remember that after a 90-degree pulse, the decay in transverse magnetization caused by dephasing due to processes intrinsic to the tissue is called T2 relaxation, and that spatial inhomogeneities in the magnetic field caused by the imperfections in the main magnet itself hastens this dephasing process; the net decrease in transverse magnetization is known as T2* (see Figs. 8-3A and B). But recall that, during

"Ideal" magnetic field

7	7	7	7	7
7	7	7	7	7
7	7	7	7	7
7	7	7	7	7
7	7	7	7	7

A

T2 relaxation

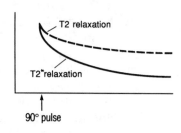

Real magnetic field

7	6	8	9	7
8	6	7	6	7
8	5	6	8	8
9	7	5	7	6
8	9	7	5	6

B

Real magnetic field with gradient

3	4	8	11	9
4	4	7	8	9
4	3	6	10	10
5	5	5	9	8
4	7	7	7	8

C

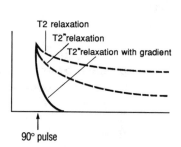

Real magnetic field with reversed gradient

11	8	8	7	3
12	8	7	4	3
12	7	6	6	4
13	9	5	5	2
12	11	7	3	2

D

Transverse magnetization

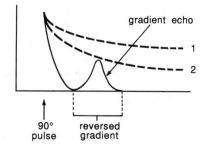

MRI processes, gradients are introduced into the main magnetic field in order to permit slice selection and image reconstruction. If any gradient is on while the transverse magnetization is relaxing, the magnetizations of the individual protons will be subjected to an additional factor, which accelerates their dephasing even more. Remember that T2 relaxation is due to variations in the magnetic field in extremely small regions which are intrinsic to the tissue and are random in time and that the additional dephasing which produces T2* decay is caused by the addition of variations in the magnetic field, which are relatively unchanging in time but which vary randomly in space. Now consider that a superimposed magnetic field gradient produces still more variation in magnetic field, which is random neither in space nor with time, but is specifically related to position in space (Fig. 8-3C). When such a gradient is applied, transverse magnetization decays even faster than T2*; the decay looks like that seen in Fig. 8-3C. Remember that a 180-degree pulse would reverse the phase of the precessing magnetizations of each proton, so that the magnetizations rephase (at least insomuch as their dephasing was due to variations in the main magnetic field rather than to true T2); a 180-degree rephasing pulse *also* rephases the portion of the dephasing that was caused by superimposed magnetic field gradients. Therefore, the amplitude of the apex of a spin

---

FIGURE 8-3.
A. The left side represents a 5 × 5 voxel slice of tissue in a perfectly homogeneous, or "ideal" magnetic field. The strength of the field in each voxel is seven arbitrary units. The right side reveals the T2 relaxation that the transverse magnetization of the tissue would undergo immediately following a 90-degree pulse. B. Real magnetic fields are inhomogeneous. On the left side, spatially random variations in the strengths of the magnetic field encountered in each voxel are seen. On the right, the T2* relaxation that would be observed after a 90-degree pulse is indicated. C. The left side reveals the real, inhomogeneous, magnetic field with a gradient superimposed. Note that in addition to the random variations in field strength, there is a general tendency for the field to become stronger as one moves from the left to the right side of the voxel array. The right side reveals the T2* relaxation that would be observed while the gradient is applied; notice that it is much steeper than the T2 relaxation or the T2* relaxation without the gradient. D. The left side reveals the strength of the magnetization in each voxel that would be seen if the direction of the gradient were reversed. The right side reveals the effect of the reversal of the gradient on the transverse magnetization. The magnetization begins to rise the instant the gradient is reversed, and continues to do so until it reaches the level of the T2* decay curve, whereupon it falls again. This signal echo is weaker than a spin echo produced by a 180-degree pulse: The apex of a spin echo would reach the level of the T2 decay curve.

echo produced by 180-degree pulse is the same whether or not a magnetic field gradient has been applied.

However, there is another way to rephase the dephasing magnetizations. Imagine that a gradient of a particular strength is applied for a particular length of time, and then that the gradient is reversed; that is, a gradient of equal amplitude (strength) but opposite direction is applied. Imagine two protons, one of which was in a relatively high field and the other of which was in a relatively low field in the original gradient. When the gradient is reversed, the one that was in a high field will then be in a relatively low field, and vice versa. Therefore, although their *phases* will not be changed by the gradient reversal, their relative *speeds* will be exchanged and they will tend to rephase. For a large population of protons, this reversal of the gradient can cause rephasing that acts in some ways like a spin echo. And since, with rephasing, the transverse magnetization grows, the emitted signal will grow as well. After the echo has reached its apex, it will die away again, since the same dephasing factors that were present earlier still persist.

The echoes produced by reversing gradients differ in several important ways from the spin echoes produced by 180-degree refocusing pulses. First of all, a 180-degree refocusing pulse transiently reverses the dephasing effect of magnetic field inhomogeneity *and* of superimposed gradients, so that the apex of the spin echo reaches the height of the T2 decay curve. But a gradient echo only reverses the dephasing effect of the gradient, not that of magnetic field inhomogeneity, so that the apex of the echo produced is only as high as the T2* decay curve (Fig. 8-3D). Therefore, all other things being equal, the amplitude of the signal of a gradient echo will be considerably smaller than that of a standard spin echo. And since the T2* decay curve falls more rapidly as magnetic field inhomogeneity gets worse, the more inhomogeneous a magnet is, the smaller will be its gradient echoes, and the worse will be the signal-to-noise ratios in the subsequent images. Since this is not a concern with standard spin echoes, spin-echo imaging can take place successfully in (relatively) inhomogeneous magnetic fields; gradient-echo imaging cannot. Another consequence of using gradient echoes instead of standard spin echoes is that the TE, which is still defined as the time between the 90-degree pulse and the appearance of the apex of the spin echo, can be made shorter than it can with standard spin echoes. A very short TE will, in part, offset the diminution in signal strength that is an inevitable consequence of using gradient echoes rather than spin echoes, and can lessen the degree to which the image is T2* weighted.

Finally, recall that the inhomogeneous distribution within tissues of substances with high magnetic susceptibility (such as methemoglobin or deoxyhemoglobin in intact red blood cells in hematomas, or ferrite particles localized within macrophages) cause local field inhomogeneities. These field inhomogeneities are corrected for by a 180-degree refocusing pulse but not by a gradient reversal. Therefore, such tissue may be represented as an even lower-signal region on gradient echo images than on standard spin-echo images.

An important feature of gradient echoes is that they *permit* small-flip-angle imaging. Pulses of 180 degrees are not usually used to form spin echoes after small-flip-angle pulses, for reasons that are easy to understand. Imagine, for example, that a tissue sample has been subjected to a 20-degree pulse. Immediately following the pulse, a large amount of longitudinal magnetization persists and a small amount of transverse magnetization has appeared. Application of a 180-degree pulse refocuses the transverse magnetization to produce a spin echo, but it also rotates the longitudinal magnetization through 180 degrees, so that a large component of longitudinal magnetization in the negative Z direction would suddenly appear. The next 20-degree pulse would act on this negative longitudinal magnetization, which would have been shrinking as a result of T1 relaxation. Then the next 180-degree pulse would flip the negative magnetization back into the positive Z direction, and so forth. Successive pulses would cause the longitudinal magnetization to flip back and forth between the positive and negative Z directions, producing a complex situation in which the size of the spin echo would vary considerably from pulse to pulse. (Indeed, even with 90-degree pulses, this phenomenon occurs, but is quantitatively unimportant.) Flipping longitudinal magnetization back and forth between the positive and negative directions by combining 180-degree refocusing pulses with small flip angles has been used to produce images with interesting contrast features, but the technique is not in common use currently.

Producing an echo using a gradient reversal does not, however, change the direction of the longitudinal magnetization at all, so that small flip angles can be used if gradient echoes are employed. It should now be clear why small flip angles and gradient echoes go hand in hand: With small flip angles, a gradient echo is necessary; conversely, with a 90-degree pulse, since a gradient echo is not necessary and since a gradient echo produces a smaller signal than does a 180-degree pulse, gradient echoes are infrequently used.

The use of gradient echoes may produce a particular kind of imaging artifact known as *magnetic susceptibility arti-*

fact. Remember that the amplitude of a gradient echo is limited by the T2* decay curve, rather than the T2 decay curve, and remember that magnetic field inhomogeneity is primarily caused by spatial variations in the strength of the main magnetic field that are produced by the magnet itself and are only partially correctable by magnetic field shimming. But spatial variations in the strength of the magnetic field may also be caused by the anatomic structure being imaged. The magnetic susceptibility of tissues, which is the degree to which the applied main magnetic field causes the tissue itself to become magnetized, differs from tissue to tissue. Therefore, at the interface between two such tissues (for example, at the junction of soft tissue and bone), there may be a relatively great local inhomogeneity. If an imaged voxel includes this interface, there will be a relatively wide range of magnetic fields within it; that is, its T2* will be extremely rapid. In this voxel, therefore, the amplitude of a gradient echo will be very small, and the voxel will appear black. And if the voxels that are occupied by such tissue interfaces all appear black, the interfaces will appear to be outlined by a thin dense black line, which constitutes one manifestation of this artifact. Alternatively, the interfaces between volumes of different magnetic susceptibilities may be much smaller. For example, hematomas in which hemoglobin has changed to deoxyhemoglobin or methemoglobin but is still contained within red blood cells may produce such field inhomogeneities, since deoxyhemoglobin and methemoglobin have a considerably higher magnetic susceptibility than plasma. These local inhomogeneities are much too small to be seen individually, of course. What happens is that the entire volume occupied by deoxyhemoglobin- or methemoglobin-containing red blood cells has considerable magnetic field inhomogeneity scattered throughout it, so the entire volume appears black (Fig. 8-4).

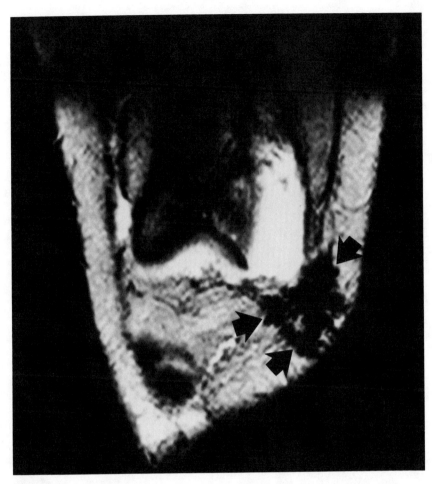

FIGURE 8-4.
Gradient-echo coronal image of a knee following arthroscopy. The irregular black region in the subcutaneous fat (arrows) represents magnetic susceptibility artifact. Focal hemosiderin deposits around the arthroscopy wound produce local inhomogeneities, which appear as a signal-free region on this T2*-weighted image. The patient had no sutures or other foreign bodies in this site.

CHAPTER 9

Flow

So far, we have seen that proton spin density, relaxation times, and pulse sequences can all affect the strength of the signal emitted by a particular portion of tissue and hence the brightness with which that tissue is displayed in the MR image. Motion of the tissue is an additional factor that may markedly alter the signal strength recorded from the moving tissue. As we have seen, certain types of motion frequently degrade the image, but the particular motion of flowing blood may be very helpful in interpreting images, since the alteration in signal intensity identifies flowing blood and thus permits identification of medium-sized and large blood vessels.

The relationship between the motion of flowing blood and the representation of the blood on images is complex; indeed, the subject of NMR flowmeters, the developing science of MRI angiography, the expanding clinical uses of blood flow signs in standard NMR imaging, and the variety of artifacts produced by blood flow comprise a body of knowledge that is largely beyond the scope of this text. We do, however, describe some of the more commonly observed flow phenomena and explain their origin.

Blood within the lumina of large vessels may have a variety of appearances on MR images. The most common is the so-called *flow void*, in which the flowing blood within vessels emits little or no signal, so that the lumina appear black (Fig. 9-1). Since this phenomenon was one of the earliest observed, when it subsequently became apparent that flowing blood might emit a relatively strong signal and appear bright, the term "paradoxical enhancement" was used, although, once understood, it became apparent that the "en-

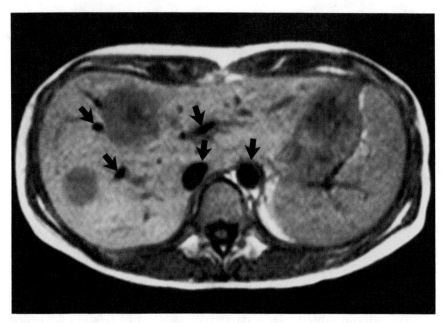

FIGURE 9-1.
Flow void. Blood moving within vessels emits negligible signal and appears black (arrows). This patient has hepatic metastatic carcinoma.

hancement" is not "paradoxical" at all. In addition, a variety of appearances of dots, rings, and streaks appearing in images of flowing blood may be encountered. Their relationship to blood flow patterns is sometimes obvious and sometimes obscure; these local flow artifacts are not dealt with here.

Two categories into which blood flow imaging phenomena can be grouped are dephasing phenomena and "time-of-flight" phenomena. We will describe each of these.

DEPHASING PHENOMENA

Imagine a very small volume of blood flowing in a vessel. It will contain a number of water molecules whose nuclei are subjected to the magnetic fields, field gradients, and radio frequency pulses described earlier for imaging experiments. Since all imaging devices involve the application of magnetic field gradients to the imaged tissue, the volume of blood will flow, at least at certain times, along gradients. Imagine that the protons have acquired some transverse magnetization in the course of the pulses that they receive. In this volume of flowing blood, no matter how small it is defined to be, the individual water molecules, and hence the protons, flow at different rates: Whether the flow is turbulent or laminar, within the volume of flowing blood there is a variety of velocities of flow. Now if the flow is through a region with a magnetic gradient (and if any component of the flow is in a direction containing a component of the gradient), the protons moving at different speeds will move up (or down) the gradient at different speeds, and thus their precessional frequencies will increase (or decrease) at different speeds. The differences in precessional frequencies among the protons are, of course, exactly the process that causes dephasing, so that the blood acts as if it has a fairly short T2, and thus emits a very small spin echo or none at all, and appears dark on images. A 180-degree refocusing pulse will not reverse the dephasing due to this particular process; for a 180-degree refocusing pulse to be effective, the differences in precessional frequencies among the protons whose magnetizations are to be refocused must be unchanging with time, which is clearly not the case with fluid flowing through gradients.

Another phenomenon that comes into play, albeit to a much lesser extent than flow within gradients, is that of magnetic field inhomogeneity. If blood flows through a field that is spatially inhomogeneous, its precessing protons will experience a field whose strength varies randomly with time, and the path of each proton will give it a unique experience of varying magnetic fields. These variations will dephase the precessing magnetizations, and, since the precessional speed differences are not constant with time, the dephased magnetizations cannot be rephased by a 180-degree pulse. Again, the effect is similar to that of shortening T2, and a subsequent loss of signal is observed.

A special circumstance may exist when blood flows in a laminar fashion along a gradient and when more than one spin echo is generated after each 90-degree pulse. Imagine that a small volume of blood is flowing in a laminar fashion along a gradient. If laminar flow conditions exist, some of the protons will consistently flow at a faster rate than others. Imagine that the protons have been subjected to a 90-degree pulse and are now precessing in the transverse plane, and imagine that they flow up a gradient. The protons that are traveling faster will, after a short period, not only be in a higher field than those flowing more slowly, but they will also be increasing the *rate* at which their ambient magnetic field—and hence their frequency—rises, faster than the fields around the slower moving protons will. Now imagine that the spins are subjected to a 180-degree pulse. Although this pulse would have rephased the spins if the spins were in different fields but stationary (that is, if their speeds of precession were different from each other but at least constant in time), if the spins are flowing at different rates, their speeds continue to change after the 180-degree pulse and, at time TE, their rephasing is not complete. Indeed, the rephasing is never complete unless a second 180-degree pulse is applied. Such a second pulse reverses the phases of the spins again. This second reversal of phases will permit the spins to rephase to the same degree they would have if they had been stationary. The resultant spin echo may be considerably stronger, therefore, than the spin echo after the first 180-degree pulse. The observed effect of all this is that if a dual-echo imaging protocol is performed, flowing blood may appear much brighter in the image with the second echo than it does in the image with the first echo (Fig. 9-2). The process can be repeated with subsequent echoes, so that the spins are dephased and flowing blood appears relatively dark in images made from the first, third, fifth, and seventh echoes, and so forth, whereas in images made from the second, fourth, sixth, and eighth echoes, and so forth, the blood appears relatively bright. True T2 decay occurs inexorably, of course, but since blood has a relatively long T2, it may appear quite bright in even echoes despite relatively long TE values. This phenomenon is known as *even-echo rephasing*.

TIME-OF-FLIGHT EFFECTS

The preceding phenomena have had to do with the dephasing of protons caused by the motion of blood within the imaging volume. Another category of flow imaging effects has to do not with dephasing, but with processes that depend on the movement of relatively large volumes of blood relative to the imaged plane; these are known as *time-of-flight effects*.

Recall that a common way to make a tomographic image is to apply a slice-selection gradient to the tissue at the same time that radio frequency pulses are applied. The frequency of the pulses and the strength of the gradient are coordinated so that the pulses affect spins only within the desired slices of tissue. The slice-selection gradient may be on both at the time the 90-degree pulse is applied and at the time the 180-degree pulse is applied. The slice thus selected will subsequently emit a spin echo that will be recorded and used to produce the image of the slice. But imagine that blood is flowing in a direction perpendicular to the slice (or at an angle such that at least some component of the flow is perpendicular to the slice). The blood within the slice at the time of the 90-degree pulse will no longer be in the slice when the 180-degree pulse is applied; instead, the lumen of

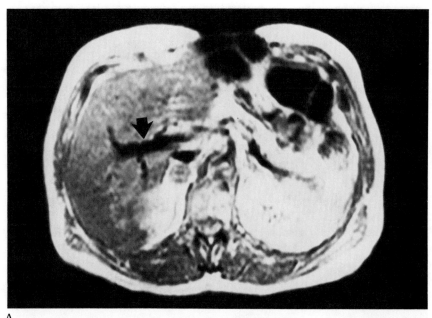

A

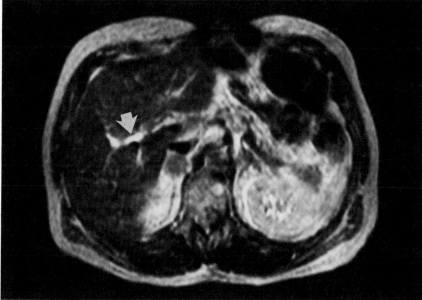

B

FIGURE 9-2.
Even-echo rephasing. The first echo (A) of this four-echo experiment shows
that moving blood (arrow) emits relatively little signal. In the image from the
second echo (B), the blood emits a stronger signal and appears brighter
(arrow).

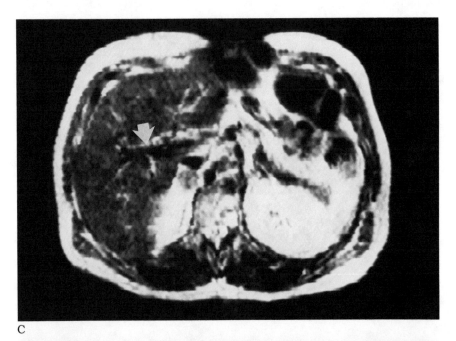

C

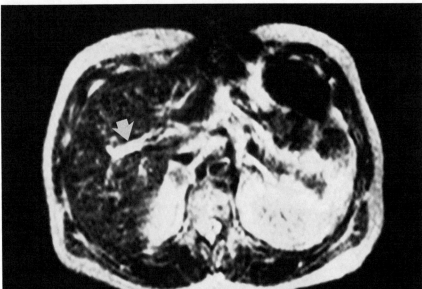

D

FIGURE 9-2 (continued).
The signal is weak (arrow) in the third-echo image (C) and strong in the
fourth-echo image (D). The stronger signals are real phenomena; they are
not just apparent increases in brightness caused by increasing the overall
gain of the image.

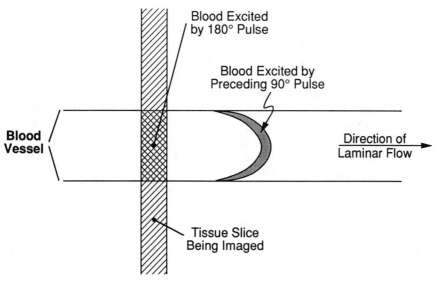

FIGURE 9-3.
A vessel containing blood with laminar flow. The slice of tissue being imaged intersects the vessel so that a disc of flowing blood is excited by each pulse. But the excited blood is carried away from the slice before a second pulse is applied. No blood is ever excited by both a 90-degree pulse and a 180-degree pulse; blood never emits a spin echo.

the blood vessel within the slice will, at the time of the 180-degree pulse, contain blood that was not in the slice at all during the 90-degree pulse, and that therefore contains no transverse magnetization (Fig. 9-3). The 180-degree pulse that affects it will therefore be unable to produce a spin echo, and the blood in the slice will emit no signal, so that the lumen of the vessel in the resulting image will appear black. The degree to which this happens depends on a number of factors, including the precise speed and direction of flow of the blood and of the TE of the pulse sequence used, but the net effect is that signal is often diminished from all or part of the blood.

A special case of the time-of-flight phenomena is called the entry-slice phenomenon. Imagine a circumstance in which blood is flowing in a vessel perpendicular to the slice of tissue being imaged. The stationary tissue in the imaged slice is subjected to a long series of 90-degree–180-degree pulse pairs. Unless TR is very long with respect to the T1 values of the stationary tissues, the longitudinal magnetization of the stationary tissue will not have undergone complete relaxation in the interval between one pulse pair and the next. Without complete regrowth of longitudinal magnetization, transverse magnetization and hence the amplitude of the spin echo will be less than the maximum possible. This is, of course, exactly the phenomenon that produces T1-dependency in the resultant images. But the flowing blood may encounter a different set of conditions. The blood within the imaged slice that is subjected to a 90-degree–180-degree pulse pair, and that subsequently emits a spin echo, may have been completely outside the imaged slice during all the preceding pulses, but may still have been within the main magnetic field for a considerable length of time. Therefore, the blood will have acquired maximum longitudinal magnetization, which will be transferred to the transverse plane by the 90-degree pulse and ultimately reflected in the magnitude of the spin echo. The imaging of the flowing blood, therefore, will not be affected by T1 processes at all, and will appear quite bright.

In a multislice imaging process (Fig. 9-4), the blood may

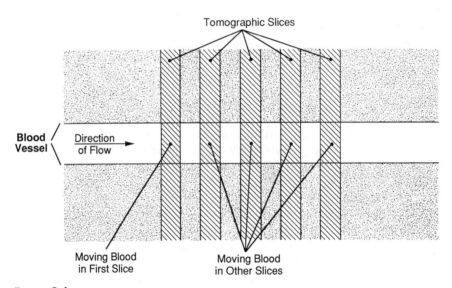

FIGURE 9-4.
Multislice imaging of a volume of tissue with a blood vessel in it; the vessel intersects all five slices. When the flow is slow enough, and TE is short enough, the phenomenon illustrated in Fig. 9-3 does not occur. However, the blood in the first slice has a unique experience: Since it has flowed from a region that is not being imaged, every pulse pair it receives is the first pulse pair to which it has been exposed; its longitudinal magnetization has not been diminished by exposure to previous pulses. However, the second, third, fourth, and fifth slices contain blood that has already been exposed in the first, second, third, or fourth slices, respectively. The longitudinal magnetization has been diminished by the pulses to which it has been exposed in slices further upstream, and therefore blood in subsequent slices emits smaller spin echoes than does the blood in the first slice.

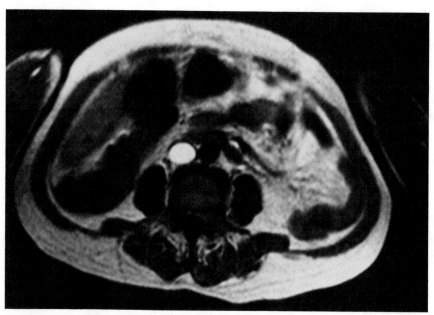

FIGURE 9-5.

Entry-slice phenomenon. This midabdominal transverse image is the most inferior of the series of slices from a multislice examination of the upper abdomen. Blood in the inferior vena cava appears very bright, since it is the first slice that blood flowing superiorly in the cava has encountered. Blood in the aorta appears quite dark, since it has encountered radio frequency pulses in more superior slices, and had its magnetization destroyed by those pulses.

appear bright only in the first slice it encounters (Fig. 9-5). As it flows from the slice at one edge of the imaging volume through other slices, the blood will be subjected to subsequent 90-degree and 180-degree pulses, and thus will never have had a chance to regain fully its longitudinal magnetization, so that in subsequent slices the blood will not form a strong spin echo and will not appear bright in the images. Thus, blood flowing into a series of tomographic images may appear bright in the first slices it encounters and darker in other slices; this is known as the *entry-slice phenomenon*. It is possible to make use of this phenomenon by imaging only a single slice at a time. Giving up multislice imaging might ordinarily require that producing many slices would take an inordinately long time, but if extremely short TR values are used, acquiring all the necessary data from one slice before going on to the next can be done relatively rapidly. Under these circumstances, each slice may act as an "entry" slice, so that blood flowing within it appears quite bright. This technique makes it possible to do a kind of tomographic MRI angiography.

If, by this time, it may seem difficult to predict exactly what sort of appearance flowing blood in a large vessel should have, do not be discouraged. Dephasing, rephasing, and time-of-flight phenomena may all operate in the same image, and produce peculiar combinations of strong signal, absent signal, peripheral signal, or central signal in vessels large enough to be seen, and it may become difficult to determine which appearances reflect flow artifacts and which appearances reflect signal from stationary tissue such as a thrombus. At the time of writing, development of pulse and gradient sequences specifically designed in order to make flowing blood appear uniformly bright or uniformly signal-free are being extensively pursued, and their state is beyond the scope of this text.

CHAPTER 10

Signal-to-Noise Issues

In MRI, maximizing signal-to-noise ratios is particularly important: The strength of the signal emitted by the imaged tissue is sufficiently low that imaging protocols must be chosen with signal strength constantly in mind, since signal-to-noise ratios are frequently low enough that the clinical utility of images is diminished. A number of parameters that control signal-to-noise ratios can be altered for every patient. This section deals with the most important of these. It should be kept in mind that signal-to-noise is not the only issue to be optimized; as we discussed in the earlier sections on pulse sequences, contrast and contrast-to-noise issues are essential as well. Nevertheless, signal-to-noise optimization is essential to perform satisfactory imaging.

NUMBER OF SPIN ECHOES

As we have seen, for standard imaging using two-dimensional Fourier transform methods, the minimum number of spin echoes that must be recorded is the same as the number of image pixels in the phase-encoding direction. However, there is no reason not to acquire more spin echoes to contribute to the total signal available to create an image. The number of spin echoes can be increased by any multiple of the original numbers to increase signal-to-noise (Fig. 10-1). There are limitations to this technique, though: The time required to collect the data for a set of images is increased linearly with the multiples used to multiply the original number of spin echoes, but the signal-to-noise ratio rises

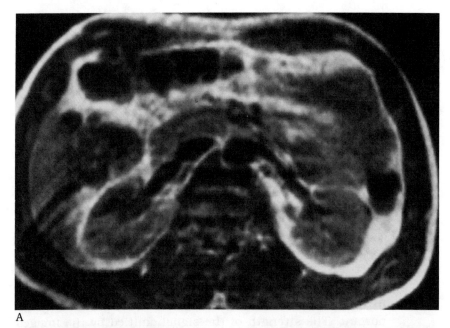

A

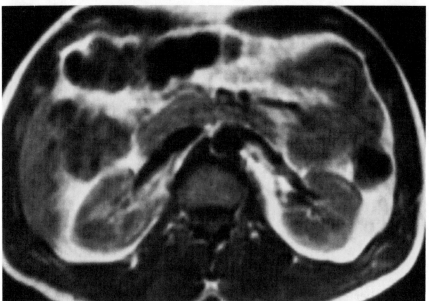

B

FIGURE 10-1.
Effect of increasing number of spin echoes. A. Only one set of spin echoes has been used. B. Four sets of spin echoes have been employed; all other factors are identical. Note the improvement in signal-to-noise.

only with the square root of that number. Real limitations are imposed by the ability of the patient to remain motionless; therefore, the longer the data are collected in order to improve the signal-to-noise ratio, the more likely the patient is to move and severely degrade the image. In addition, there is an interplay between TR and the number of measurements that can be made: The longer the TR, the longer a single group of spin echoes will require, and the fewer groups of measurements will be permitted within a given imaging time. Also, the greater the number of pixels in the phase-encoding direction, the greater the number of spin echoes that will be required, and the fewer the number of groups of measurements that can be made.

The imaging devices from different manufacturers use different terminologies to describe each group of measurements. Each group of the minimum number of spin echoes may be known as an *acquisition*, a *measurement*, or an *average*. Other terminology calls the summing of *two* sets of spin echoes as one "average." It is common to use two to four groups of spin echoes when TR values are relatively short, and one or two groups of spin echoes when TR values are relatively long, although these numbers may be varied considerably in practice.

VOXEL SIZE

Since tissue emits both the signal and some of the noise that contribute to an image, if one considers a single voxel, it should be obvious that the more voluminous the voxel, the stronger the signal will be. Voxel volume can be increased in several ways.

The first method is to increase the slice thickness (Fig. 10-2). If the slice thickness doubles, the voxel volume will double and the signal-to-noise ratio will also double. This improvement comes at a price, of course; the thicker the slice, the worse are problems encountered with partial volume averaging and the less distinct will be most borders between different tissues.

The next method is to increase the area, or field of view, of each image. If, for example, the dimension of each image is increased by two both in the phase-encoding and frequency-encoding directions, the area of the entire image will be increased by a factor of four, and hence the volume of each voxel, and the signal strength, will also be increased by a factor of four (Fig. 10-3). But, as so often turns out to be true, this improvement does not come free either:

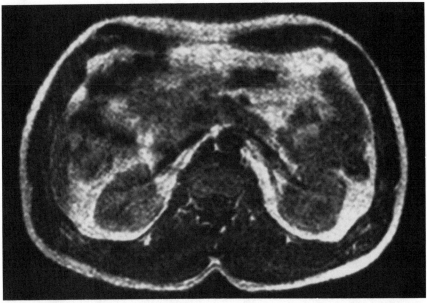

A

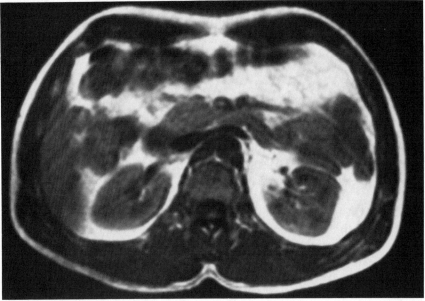

B

FIGURE 10-2.
Effect of increasing slice thickness. A. Three-millimeter slice. B. Ten-millimeter slice. Factors other than the slice thickness are identical. Note the increased signal-to-noise in the thicker slice.

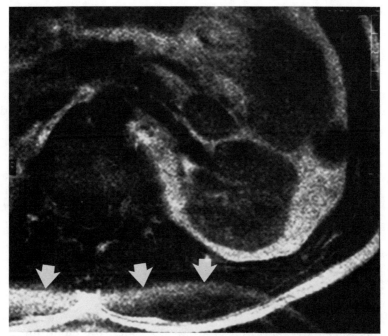

A

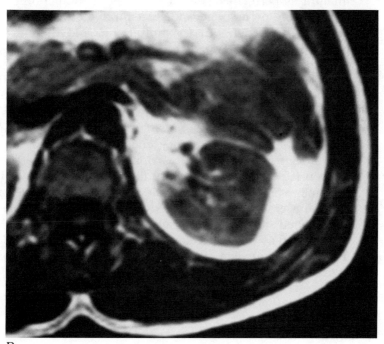

B

FIGURE 10-3.
Effect of increasing field of view. A. Small field of view. A wraparound artifact
(arrows), caused by the appearance of anterior subcutaneous fat, is seen.
B. Large field of view. Other factors have been held constant, and the magni-
fication of the two images has been altered so that the structures appear
with similar dimensions. Note the increased signal-to-noise in the large field
of view image.

The increased voxel size tends to cause a diminution in the spatial resolution of the image.

Alternatively, the field of view may be kept constant but the number of pixels in the overall array may be diminished. The size of each pixel therefore increases by a corresponding factor, the volume of each voxel increases by the same factor (assuming a constant slice thickness), and the signal-to-noise ratio in each pixel goes up; again, loss of spatial resolution tends to occur. If the number of pixels in the phase-encoding direction is decreased, the number of required spin echoes will also diminish, with a consequent decrease in imaging time.

SLICE GAP

In a previous section, we discussed how narrow or absent slice gaps tend to accentuate T1 weighting when multislice imaging is performed. Recall that this phenomenon occurs because radio frequency pulses cannot be produced with precisely defined frequency limitations, and therefore the pulses that are intended to affect only one slice of tissue tend to affect nearby tissue as well. Remember that the time between successive 90-degree pulses intended for a particular slice is TR, and that this interval is the time during which the longitudinal magnetization of each slice is regained during the process of T1 relaxation. But if, during this interval, radio frequency energy intended for an adjacent slice affects the slice's longitudinal magnetization while it is relaxing, that longitudinal magnetization will be, to some extent, diminished. The magnetization moved into the transverse plane by the next 90-degree pulse will also be diminished, and the signal arising from that slice will be diminished as well. Therefore, it is advisable to leave at least a small gap between slices in order to avoid reductions in signal-to-noise.

ECHO TIME

As we discussed in previous sections, T2 decay causes the strength of each spin echo to diminish as TE gets longer; there is, of course, a consequent loss in signal-to-noise. The magnitude of this loss varies from tissue to tissue.

REPETITION TIME

As TR lengthens, each tissue's maximum longitudinal magnetization tends to increase, and hence the strength of the spin echo increases as well. The consequent improvement in signal-to-noise is limited: Once complete longitudinal relaxation has occurred for a given tissue, no additional improvement can be expected with increasing TR.

INVERSION TIME

In inversion recovery images, TI also affects signal-to-noise, but in a more complex way than does TR and TE. If TI is very short, longitudinal magnetization is still inverted at the time of a 90-degree pulse, yielding a large signal. As it increases, the weaker the signal will be and the smaller the signal-to-noise ratio will be. As TI continues to increase beyond the point at which a given tissue's longitudinal magnetization has crossed the zero point, the longer the TI, the stronger the signal-to-noise will be. TI values that give high signal-to-noise ratios tend to produce relatively low image contrast, and vice versa. This unfortunate trade-off is also true of TE and TR.

SURFACE COILS

Earlier in the text, we mentioned that the radio frequency signal emitted by tissue is detected by monitoring the alternating voltage induced in antennae wires near the patients. We mentioned that these coils may be used also to transmit the radio frequency pulses that are applied to the patient, or that separate coils may transmit the radio frequency pulses, and that the radio frequency emitted by the tissue may be detected using "receive-only" coils.

Receiving coils need to be designed and positioned so that they are maximally sensitive to emitted radio frequency signals, that is, so that they have the largest possible voltage induced in them by the radio frequency signal emitted by the tissue. This requires that the wires of the coil be as close to the imaged tissues as possible. It also requires that as much of the space as possible within the coil be filled by the tissue being imaged. We do not intend to go into the configuration of these coils, but do wish to point out that they fall into two main categories, the so-called surface coils and the more standard shapes.

The standard designs are usually configured as "head" or "body" coils. Each is shaped so that their wires travel within a form usually shaped like the surface of a short cylinder. Body coils have a relatively large diameter and contain the chest, abdomen, or pelvis of most adults. Head coils are of appropriate diameter to contain an adult head, but they can equally well be used to examine the trunks of small children. Indeed, of the standard coils, the smaller should be used whenever possible, since smaller body parts will fill the central portions of such coils better and be closer to the wires of the coil, which, as we mentioned, are situations that increase the voltage induced in the wires.

Standard head and body coils are designed so that, as much as possible, radio frequency signal emitted from tissue anywhere within them will induce voltage that does not vary depending on whether the voxel emitting the signal is near the periphery of the body in the coil wire or deep within the imaged volume and thus far from the wire. If a coil design fails to demonstrate this uniformity of spatial sensitivity, the resultant images would have darker and lighter regions within them, which would greatly complicate the interpretation of their contrast.

Incidentally, the coils that emit the radio frequency pulses are designed similarly: As much as possible, they deliver the same strength of radio frequency energy to all voxels within their imaging volume. If they failed to do so, radio frequency pulses that constituted 90- or 180-degree pulses for some voxels would flip the tissues' net magnetizations more or less than 90 or 180 degrees in other voxels, which would, in turn, considerably alter the strength of the spin echoes emitted from those voxels, and produce artifactual alterations in image contrast.

Surface coils, on the other hand, are usually not embedded in cylindrical surfaces but rest within flat, slightly curved, or malleable containers and are placed directly on the skin. These are usually used to image structures relatively close to the surface of the body. By virtue of being closer to the tissue that emits the signal, and by having a quite small amount of their internal space filled with air, the surface coils are, in general, more sensitive than standard coils, and their greater voltage permits an image with a relatively high signal-to-noise ratio (Fig. 10-4). But this increased sensitiv-

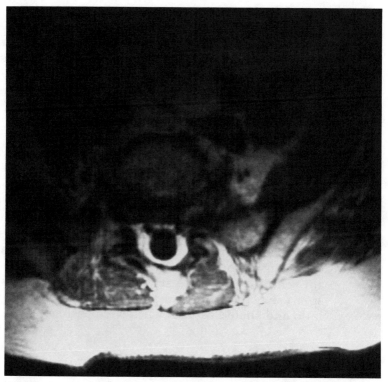

FIGURE 10-4.
Effect of surface coil. Notice the increased signal-to-noise ratio in the body parts near the surface. The signal strength falls off rapidly for deeper structures, however.

ity comes at a cost: They usually do *not* receive signal from all the imaged voxels with the same sensitivity. In general, the farther the tissue is from the coil, the less its emitted signal is received by the coil, so that images produced with these coils tend to appear brightest in regions near the coil and progressively darker in regions remote from the coil. To some degree, this signal fall-off can be compensated for, but, as one might imagine, it makes estimation of the true signal strength of a particular anatomic region difficult, and also makes imaging of deep structures unsatisfactory.

CHOICE OF FLIP ANGLE

In the discussion of small flip angles, we explained that only a small amount of a tissue's longitudinal magnetization is moved into the transverse plane if a small flip angle is used. Thus there is less transverse magnetization available to produce radio frequency signal from the tissue. The relationships among flip angles, TR values, T1s, and signal strength are complex, but, in general (and all other things being equal), an extremely small flip angle will produce a relatively low signal-to-noise value.

CHOICE OF ECHO TYPE

Recall from an earlier discussion that a gradient echo has the apex of its envelope reach the amplitude that the T2* decay curve (or FID) would have been in the absence of gradients, whereas a spin echo produced by a 180-degree refocusing pulse will have the apex of its envelope reach the T2 decay curve. Therefore, all other things being equal, a gradient echo will produce a smaller signal than will a standard spin echo; the latter will produce a higher signal-to-noise ratio and should be used whenever possible.

Afterword

We hope that by now you have gained an understanding of the basic principles that underlie magnetic resonance imaging. We have discussed the major physical phenomena involved in MRI; the major operations each MRI device performs when examining patients; how to alter imaging parameters to affect image contrast, signal-to-noise ratio, and imaging time; and the characteristics of tissues implied by their imaging appearance. Armed with this information, you should be able to experiment with and modify your own imaging protocols to optimize them for your particular scanner and clinical practice, and you should often be able to decipher puzzling images when you encounter them. Finally, you should now be equipped to understand advances in MRI as the technology evolves. Good luck!

J.H.N.
J.I.W.

Index